T0250056

Tackling Health Inequalities

Although environmental health has received some recognition as a field which can positively impact on the social determinants of health, it remains little known outside its immediate sphere of influence. There is also limited literature available to support the potential impact of the profession in public health policy circles, and there has been an overreliance on anecdotal rather than firm evidence.

This book presents the findings of an empirical research project focussed on public health policymaking (English Health and Wellbeing Boards), health inequalities and environmental health and provides an insight to the environmental health profession and routes of impact and influence. It discusses environmental health in the context of public health, the role of the profession, issues of visibility and opportunities for impact in today's policy landscape. In particular, a focus on the local government context is timely given the shift of the public health function from the National Health Service to local authorities. This book is essential reading for students, practitioners and policymakers in the fields of environmental health and public health.

Surindar Dhesi is a lecturer and course leader of the MSc Science of Occupational Health, Safety and Environment at the University of Birmingham. She is also an active Chartered Environmental Health Practitioner and is a Fellow of the Higher Education Academy.

Routledge Focus on Environmental Health
Series editor: Stephen Battersby, MBE, PhD, FCIEH, FRSPH

Pioneers in Public Health
Lessons from History
Edited by Jill Stewart

Tackling Health Inequalities
Reinventing the Role of Environmental Health
Surindar Dhesi

Tackling Health Inequalities
Reinventing the Role of
Environmental Health

Surindar Dhesi

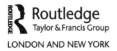

Routledge
Taylor & Francis Group

LONDON AND NEW YORK

First published 2019
by Routledge
2 Park Square, Milton Park, Abingdon, Oxon OX14 4RN

and by Routledge
52 Vanderbilt Avenue, New York, NY 10017

*Routledge is an imprint of the Taylor & Francis Group, an informa
business*

British Library Cataloguing-in-Publication Data
A catalogue record for this book is available from the
British Library

Library of Congress Cataloging-in-Publication Data
Names: Dhesi, Surindar, author.
Title: Tackling health inequalities: reinventing the role of
environmental health / Surindar Dhesi.
Description: First edition. | Abingdon, Oxon: Routledge, 2019. |
Series: Routledge focus on environmental health |
Includes bibliographical references.
Identifiers: LCCN 2018038905 | ISBN 9781138095748 (hardback) |
ISBN 9781315105598 (ebook)
Subjects: LCSH: Environmental health. | Environmental justice. |
Pollution—Health aspects. | Public health. | Medical policy—England.
Classification: LCC RA565 .D45 2019 | DDC 613/.1—dc23
LC record available at https://lccn.loc.gov/2018038905

ISBN: 978-1-138-09574-8 (hbk)
ISBN: 978-1-315-10559-8 (ebk)

Typeset in Times New Roman
by codeMantra

For my students and their students

Contents

Figures and tables

Figures

Tables

Series preface

This new series, Routledge Focus on Environmental Health, aims to explore environmental health topics and issues in more detail than might be found in the usual environmental health texts. As part of this we want to encourage readers and practitioners, particularly those who might not have had work published previously, to submit proposals as we hope to be responsive to the needs of environmental and public health practitioners. I am keen that this is seen as an opportunity for first-time authors. This is a dynamic series, which aims to provide a forum for new ideas and debate on current environmental health topics. So it is an exciting development for environmental and public health practitioners, particularly for new professionals. So if you have any ideas for monographs in the series please do not be afraid to submit them to me as series editor via the e-mail address below.

I have always encouraged new authors and for environmental health practitioners on the front line to "get published" writing from their experiences of trying to protect public health – putting down in writing an analysis of what worked, what was successful what wasn't and why, can provide useful insights for others working in the field. Furthermore, why for example should the hard work that has gone into a dissertation lie in an unread book on a library shelf? All too often the work of EHPs goes unrecorded and unremarked and with the demise of the Journal of Environmental Health I am pleased to be working with Routledge to provide this opportunity to provide another route for practitioners to change this.

The initiative for this series followed from the publication of the 21st Edition of Clay's Handbook of Environmental Health in July 2016, but that is largely a technical work and first point of reference. It is not intended that this series takes a wholly "technical" approach but provides an opportunity to consider areas of practice in a different way, for example looking at the social and political aspects of environmental health in addition to a more discursive approach on specialist areas.

We recognise that "environmental health" can be taken to mean different things in different countries around the World. I know that Clay's has chapters that might not be relevant to some practitioners in different countries, nevertheless EHPs are a key part of the public health workforce wherever they practise. So, this series will enable a wider range of practitioners and others with a professional interest to access information and also to write about issues relevant to them. The format means a relatively short production time so contents will be more immediate than in a standard textbook or reference work.

Forthcoming monographs are likely to cover such areas as Housing and Health, Dealing with environmental health problems associated with residential property, and Air pollution and health. That does not mean we have no need of further suggestions, quite the contrary, so I hope readers with ideas for a monograph will get in touch via Ed.Needle@tandf.co.uk.

Foreword

This book is essential reading for all who work in, or value the work of, environmental health practitioners. It is particularly relevant to those responsible for the design and delivery of public health policy at strategic level, because it sets out the case for recognising and valuing a significant element of the workforce which the author identifies as 'invisible'. At this time of crisis of affordability in our National Health Service and increasing inequalities in health, it cannot be acceptable that such an important resource is not fully engaged and utilised.

I have known Surindar for many years and have been a champion for her work. She identifies her doctorate thesis, *Exploring how Health and Wellbeing Boards are tackling health inequalities with particular reference to the role of environmental health*, as the trigger for this exposition of a profession with a long history but one which urgently needs to examine its impact and influence in these times of austerity in our public services and endless, unaffordable demands on our health services. This publication has both practical and academic applications and should be recognised as a call to action.

For my own generation, there has never been any doubt that all of us who work in environmental health are also delivering public health improvements and reducing health inequalities and that we should therefore be properly identified as part of the public health workforce. Indeed, my own initial qualification was as a public health inspector, and I worked alongside those other professionals responsible for maintaining and improving health at the community level, including such lost titles as community health physicians, geriatric health visitors and community development officers.

The collaborative approach we environmental health professionals provided included information and advice as well as the maintenance and, where necessary, enforcement of statutory standards designed to safeguard health by mitigating the effects of the environment on human health and the transmission of infections and avoidance of accidental injury. Surindar correctly identifies this as working 'upstream', and it is an essential element of improving the quality of life and reducing demands on care and treatment services.

People's health should not be defined by their social class, and our life paths are not fixed. We can eliminate or mitigate environmental hazards to health, and we can also create environments conducive to good health and make the healthier choices the easier choices. No country can consider that it provides a comprehensive health service if it neglects to invest in the prevention of ill health and the reduction of health inequalities. This approach requires the contributions of environmental health practitioners, and this book provides us with the all the information we need to make the case for gaining proper recognition of environmental health practice and to call for revitalising the profession.

Surindar takes the call for action further and requires that we reinvent environmental health to be fit for the public health challenges of the future. The actions she identifies are the means to do this, and her personal example can be our motivation.

Ian Gray, MBE
Associate Director
Environmental Health Collaborating Centre

Acknowledgements

With thanks to Dr Anna Coleman, Professor Kath Checkland and Professor Stephen Harrison for their kindness and guidance during and since my time at the University of Manchester. Professor Harrison passed away during the editing of this book and his loss is sorely felt.

Thanks also to Zena Lynch and Professor Roy Harrison for their trust and commitment to academic freedom at the University of Birmingham.

Thank you to my students, who engaged with these ideas and helped me think through and sharpen them. In particular, to Muhammad Nasir and Mitoriana Porusia in Indonesia, Alaa Fadlallah and Matthew Kure in Nigeria, Ibrahim Al Miari in Lebanon and Salma Al Zadjali in Oman, all inspirational in their own ways. I am so proud of you and grateful for the lessons gently taught.

Finally, thank you to my editor, Dr Stephen Battersby, for his patience and practical assistance in making this monograph a reality.

1 Introduction

Environmental health as a profession has a long history of taking action to protect the public from illness and accident in the home, workplace and elsewhere. Environmental health is a specialism of public health, and practitioners are often employed in local authority regulatory roles, although an increasing number work in the private sector. The regulatory role sets it apart from other public health occupations, as practitioners can serve legal notices and take prosecution action to enforce change where necessary. The focus of this book is on environmental health in this local authority context.

Environmental health activities are geared towards the prevention of harm and providing the conditions for citizens to live healthy and long lives. These actions tend to be structural, dealing with the causes of issues, and are thus known as 'upstream' interventions, in comparison to 'downstream' interventions, which are based on alleviating the effects of adverse impacts rather than preventing them occurring.

The outcomes of upstream interventions and actions can be difficult to measure and sometimes will only be felt in the long term, in some cases taking many years to secure health improvements. Such actions, particularly if regulatory, may cause inconvenience and expense with no immediately visible result and so can be unpopular with individuals, communities and even with government. Thus, a career in environmental health can be challenging as well as rewarding!

Health inequalities are one of the most pressing public health issues we face globally and are particularly acute in countries with neoliberal economies and large societal inequalities, such as the UK and the US (Wilkinson and Pickett 2010; Schrecker and Bambra 2015). The term describes differences in health (both morbidity and mortality) between people in different socio-economic groups, with longer lives and better health experienced by people in higher socio-economic positions (Marmot and Wilkinson 2006; Marmot 2010).

In 'The Health Divide', Margaret Whitehead offers a useful definition, including the concept of fairness in relation to tackling inequalities:

> In health terms, ideally everyone should have a fair opportunity to attain their full health potential and, more pragmatically, none should be disadvantaged from achieving this potential if it can be avoided.
>
> (Whitehead 1988: 222)

And the link to social justice, equity and the resultant moral imperative for action has remained important for many working in this area, including myself.

The differences in morbidity and mortality apply at all levels in society, and we now know that having large gaps between the socio-economic status of different groups in society is detrimental not only to the people at the bottom but also to those at the top. This is thought to be related to the stress associated with either maintaining a level of status and material wealth or in feeling of diminished value if this is not achievable (Wilkinson and Pickett 2018).

Although the UK has measured, monitored and researched health inequalities for longer than any other country (Mackenbach 2010), they have remained stubbornly persistent despite various policy initiatives (Bartley 2017). This failure has been acknowledged by the central government:

> Health inequalities between rich and poor have been getting progressively worse. We still live in a country where the wealthy can expect to live longer than the poor.
>
> (Department of Health 2010)

However, there appears to be a reluctance at a high level to acknowledge and act upon the established links between health inequalities and other societal inequalities, including economic and power disparities, and how these intersect between different population groups.

Health and societal inequalities are complex and intractable and are also known as 'wicked' issues (Hunter, Marks et al. 2010), as the causes are multiple and far from straightforward to address and in some cases not fully understood. Nevertheless, even in the face of little or no progress, there is an ethical imperative to take action, since health inequalities represent a great deal of avoidable suffering (Marmot 2010). To illustrate, there is a 28-year gap in life expectancy between wealthy and deprived areas in one Scottish city (Marmot 2015).

An important but often unrecognised aspect of the environmental health role is the effect of upstream interventions tackling the 'causes of the causes' of health inequalities, also known as the 'social determinants' of health. Environmental health practitioners hold a key position in being able to take effective, enforceable action to tackle some of the causes of health inequalities at a local level and, with coordinated effort, to impact morbidity and mortality at a national population level, too.

Interventions such as improving privately rented housing stock, dealing with air, water and land pollution, protecting people from illness and injury at work and ensuring safe food and water all make a significant contribution to protecting the public's health. Nevertheless, the potential of the work to tackle health inequalities is often overlooked by people both within and outside the profession.

Chris Day sums up the imperative for environmental health practitioners to protect the most vulnerable members of society who are not in a position to improve their own circumstances:

> we should recognise where the gaps exist ... and then do something ourselves to fill it ... [because] as a group of front-line professionals we encounter in our daily round most, if not all, of the stressors that impact on human health, and driven by a desire to better the lot of those dealt a poor hand from the start, challenge the environmental service to deliver to the needs of those who may not have the capacity to speak up for themselves.
>
> (Day 2011: 64)

This statement alludes to societal inequalities impacting those affected by being in lower socio-economic positions across the course of their lives; these are deeply connected to inequalities in health. Whilst tackling the causes of health inequalities crosses the remit of many professional groups and cannot be addressed by one group alone (and certainly not only the healthcare services), environmental health has a significant potential to alleviate suffering and to address the immediate causes, and the causes of the causes, of ill health and accidents.

As an environmental health practitioner, there have been many situations where I have taken action to protect people who are unable to resolve matters themselves, for example, in improving workplace conditions, ensuring good food hygiene, dealing with noise and odour pollution and addressing unsafe housing. Over many years, I noted the quiet but important work of practitioners, hidden behind the scenes, was often unrecognised and siloed, taking place in isolation from other public health practitioners with similar goals and aspirations. Thus, when I began my PhD looking at local policies aimed at tackling health inequalities, it was important to me to include a focus on my own profession, and I am grateful to my supervisory team for supporting this decision and to my fellow practitioners for their openness, making the research possible.

My research looked at newly established English local government-based public health policymaking structures called Health and Wellbeing Boards, focusing on four case study sites in the Midlands and North. In addition, I spoke to environmental health practitioners and managers at 15 additional sites across the country, interviewing 50 people in total. I also looked at the documents produced by the boards and observed meetings over a 12-month period. Case study site descriptions are given in Table 1.1, and additional site descriptions are given in Table 1.2.

Table 1.1 Case study site numbers and descriptions

Case study site	Description	Unitary/ Upper-tier council
1	Midlands, suburban and rural areas, affluent with North-South split in areas of deprivation. The population is both growing (rising birth rate) and ageing, and 90% describe themselves as 'white British'. There are concerns around dementia, hospice provision and carers. Unemployment levels are falling, although youth unemployment remains an issue.	Upper-tier
2	Midlands, suburban and rural areas surrounding a major multicultural city, primarily affluent but with pockets of deprivation. There is a growing and ageing population, and the number of people below pension age is lower than the UK average. Ninety per cent describe themselves as 'white British'.	Upper-tier
3	Midlands, urban, with significant areas of deprivation and a 'young' population (almost half are under 30) which is very ethnically diverse, with 90% of people in some wards describing themselves as other than 'white British'. Suburbs are generally affluent, and inner-city population density is high. Air quality is often poor, and there are concerns about obesity, particularly in children.	Unitary
4	North West, urban and suburban with significant areas of deprivation. The population is ageing and almost 97% describe themselves as 'white British'. Life expectancy is lower than the national average. Smoking, drinking and substance misuse are concerns.	Unitary

Table 1.2 Additional site numbers and descriptions

Additional site	Description	Unitary/district or borough council
5	Mixed rural and suburban area, very affluent (South East)	District
6	National policymaker	N/A
7	Mainly rural county, with pockets of deprivation and affluence (South West)	Unitary
8	Mainly rural area, with pockets of deprivation and affluence (North West)	District
9	Mixed urban and suburban area (South Central)	Borough
10	Mainly rural area, with pockets of deprivation and affluence (South West)	District
11	Mainly urban and suburban with several areas of deprivation (North East)	Unitary
12	Mainly urban and suburban, very affluent area (South East)	Borough
13	Environmental Health academic	N/A
14	Mainly urban and suburban with several areas of deprivation (North West)	Unitary
15	Mainly rural area, with pockets of deprivation and affluence (East of England)	District
16	Mainly urban and suburban with several areas of deprivation (South West)	Unitary
17	Mainly urban and suburban with several areas of deprivation (Yorkshire and Humber)	Unitary
18	Mixed rural and suburban area, with pockets of significant deprivation (South East)	District
19	Urban, very affluent (London)	Unitary

At the additional sites, I focused on environmental health services, and a range of unitary, district and borough councils were selected for inclusion across a wide geographical area. The Table 1.2 shows the site numbers, provides a short description of the area and the structure.

Health and Wellbeing Boards became operational in 2013 and are (amongst other things) charged with tackling health inequalities in their local areas and designed to bring together high-level policymakers across local authorities and health services. They are required to carry out a Joint Strategic Needs Assessment of local health needs and to develop Joint Health and Wellbeing Strategies to address those needs. The idea is that the agreed policies are then followed by commissioners of services in a coherent and joined-up way with the aim of improving the health of the local population. A list of statutory members was provided by central government, with a focus on elected members, directors of public health, representatives of adults' and children's services and healthcare services, but did not include environmental health representatives, and I was interested in how my profession would fare in these arrangements.

Whilst the focus of the research was on one type of policymaking arrangement, it has generated helpful insights into how the health inequalities are being understood and tackled and how environmental health fits into the narrative at a strategic level. For this reason, and also for the benefit and ease of readers outside the English system, I have in general referred to Health and Wellbeing Boards as 'public health policymaking groups' and their members as 'public health policymakers'.

This book is the product of my experience as a practitioner, researcher and lecturer. Across these interconnected roles, I have found that the potential of environmental health in tackling health inequalities has been largely unrecognised by the wider public health workforce, but also by many environmental health practitioners.

This experience has led to a strong desire to encourage environmental health practitioners to grasp the opportunities available and to explicitly define their role as one of addressing social, environmental and health injustices and inequalities. We need to claim a policy space beyond the technical expertise for which we are currently (rightly) recognised, and for this to happen, we need a workforce that understands and can speak the language of health services and public health and that uses the available evidence and contributes to the base of knowledge on what does and doesn't work.

In Chapter 2, I introduce the environmental health profession, including the historic context and development of the role as it is today from the original inspectors of nuisances. This is followed by a discussion of the impact of environmental health on social determinants of health by upstream interventions and then an analysis of the profession as it is today.

In Chapter 3, the focus is on health inequalities. I start by considering the causes and discussing how they could be tackled with a focus on the opportunities offered, moving on to the various understandings of health inequalities expressed by public health policymakers and finally considering actions to tackle health inequalities with reference to the potential contribution of environmental health.

Chapter 4 covers public health policymaking, starting by setting out the new English structures and introducing evidence from my research across four case study sites. The policymaking process and its impacts in terms of approaches to tackling health inequalities are discussed in relation to Harrison's 'Design to Doodle' concept. Finally, the impact of politics in public health policymaking is considered in the local government context.

In Chapter 5, my research findings which revealed the invisibility of the environmental health profession are presented; this is followed by a discussion of understandings of environmental health by other members of the public health community. Challenges and suggestions for becoming more visible are considered.

Chapter 6 considers the future of environmental health in the wider public health context. I discuss perceptions of different professional groups as 'thinkers' and 'doers', the role of evidence-based practice and the need for strong links and overlaps between practitioners and their academic colleagues. Finally, strategies for increasing the impact of the profession are discussed.

The Conclusion pulls together the findings across the chapters and makes recommendations for action to reinvent environmental health so as to be fit for the public health challenges of the future.

Although the data on which this book is based was collected in England, I hope that the principles and ideas discussed resonate with my colleagues across the world, since we share common hopes and aims even if our daily circumstances and the technical nature of our challenges may differ. Health inequalities are most definitely a global phenomenon, and we can learn much from our international friends and colleagues.

References

Bartley, M. (2017). *Health Inequality: An Introduction to Theories, Concepts and Methods*. Cambridge, Polity Press.

Day, C. (2011). "Environmental Health – its practice and promotion." In *Clay's Handbook of Environmental Health*. Ed. S. Battersby. London, Routledge: 51–84.

Department of Health (2010). *Healthy Lives, Healthy People: Our Strategy for Public Health in England*. Department of Health. London, HMSO.

Hunter, D. J., L. Marks, and K. E. Smith (2010). *The Public Health System in England*. Bristol, Policy Press.

Mackenbach, J. P. (2010). "Has the English strategy to reduce health inequalities failed?" *Social Science and Medicine* 71: 1249–1253.

Marmot, M. (2010). *Fair Society, Healthy Lives: Strategic Review of Health Inequalities in England post 2010*. London, UCL.

Marmot, M. (2015). *The Health Gap*. London, Bloomsbury.

Marmot, M. and R. Wilkinson (2006). *Social Determinants of Health*. Oxford, Oxford University Press.

Schrecker, T. and C. Bambra (2015). *How Politics Makes Us Sick. Neoliberal Epidemics.* Basingstoke, Palgrave Macmillan.

Whitehead, M. (1988). *The Health Divide.* Harmondsworth, Penguin.

Wilkinson, R. and K. Pickett (2010). *The Spirit Level: Why Equality Is Better for Everyone.* London, Penguin Books.

Wilkinson, R. and K. Pickett (2018). *The Inner Level.* London, Allen Lane.

2 Environmental health as a public health profession

The historic role and context

Public health medicine in England has historically spanned the health services and local government, with local authority-based medical officers of health and their sanitary inspector assistants working together as long ago as the mid-1800s (Betts 1993; Hamlin 2013).

Initially, the role and remuneration were rather bleak, as a president of The Sanitary Inspectors Association describes:

> It was soon found by experience that the medical officer of health required a working hand, since it was impossible for him to go from his office to inspect every danger to health. In this way sprang up the sanitary inspector .... His duties were laborious, his salary contemptible. I designated him, in his first days, as the Forlorn Hope of Sanitation.
>
> (Johnson cited by Betts 1993: 47)

These sanitary inspectors were formerly known as inspectors of nuisances (Hatchett, Spear et al. 2012; Hamlin 2013) and later as public health inspectors, before becoming environmental health officers or practitioners, as they are currently called. The common thread through these various iterations has been a focus on preventing ill health and accidents resulting from environmental factors connected with living and working conditions.

Public health, including the environmental health specialism, was based in local authorities until a large reorganisation in 1974 (Griffiths 2003). This controversial restructuring split the public health professions, moving part of the workforce to the health service and leaving environmental health in local authorities (Allen 1991). Importantly, social workers, planners, leisure services and several other professional groups with remits impacting the wider determinants of health remained in local authorities. The Parliamentary Select Committee on Health (2001) summed up the detail and some of the adverse and perhaps unforeseen consequences of the reorganisation:

> The post of Medical Officer of Health was abolished in 1974 and the responsibility for monitoring environmental determinants of health passed to Directors of Environmental Health who were employed by local authorities. Doctors trained in public health medicine became Community Medicine Specialists employed by health authorities to monitor the health status of the population and advise health authorities on how best to tackle the health problems of their community. Before 1974, the Medical Officer of Health had responsibility for the provision of some personal health services and in addition, was able to influence, as an officer of the local authority, social and environmental aspects of health. These functions were lost as a result of the transfer of the Medical Officer of Health into the Health Service ....
>
> (House of Commons Select Committee on Health 2001: 27)

The new arrangements thus compromised the ability of environmental health practitioners to work as a team with medical doctors specialising in public health to take action on the determinants of health in their areas, and this was recognised by policymakers as part of the later reorganisation which is discussed in this book.

As I have described, prior to 1974, medical officers of health were administratively responsible for sanitary inspectors and this had unfortunate consequences in that 'the initial disparity in status and education between the medical officers of health and the nuisance officers sowed the seeds of rivalry and resentment' (Cornell 1996: 74). Following the 1974 reorganisation, this separation and disconnect of the disciplines has increased over the years, as MacGibbon, chairman of the Environmental Health Commission, pointed out; 'health' and 'environment' have 'drifted apart, both conceptually and in our institutions' (MacGibbon 1997: 2). She noted at that time that health policy has tended to focus on treating ill health, whilst environmental policy has broadened and, at times, moved away from health issues; others agreed, noting that environmental health and National Health Service (NHS Public Health) departments had very little contact (Cornell 1996).

The Environmental Health Commission (1997: 3) concluded that the divergence between medicine and environment needed to be reversed in recognition of the wider determinants of health and went on to recommend that environmental health and public health be linked again at a local level and better coordinated at higher levels. Around ten years before the commission, Lewis (1986) had identified an absence of a clear philosophy and direction in public health. In the 1980s, the 'new' public health movement emerged which focused on the social determinants of health, recognising that the role of the medical professions in improving public health is limited and expensive, and also noting the role of 'environmental factors' on health (Ashton and Seymour 1988). Green and Thorogood cite Action and Chambers, who said

> this is not without irony for the present day environmental health officers, who feel that this is what they have been saying and doing all along, but without the benefit of either a medical degree's status or indeed its salary!
>
> (Green and Thorogood 1998: 32)

Twenty-five years ago, Betts (1993: 129) described environmental health as the local government 'service department which is most closely associated with health … Almost all of its duties have an impact upon health'. The duties have not significantly changed in the intervening years, and recognition of the health role remains patchy. He noted that environmental health had not 'developed an independent and critical voice or developed a wider role' and said that this was partly because of government restrictions both at central and local levels. He also noted that the profession had not risen to its potential in tackling health inequalities and had failed to take the necessary strategic role in health promotion.

Today, environmental health encompasses a wide range of functions, and the World Health Organization (WHO) definition is a good reference point in describing the contemporary role:

> Environmental health addresses all the physical, chemical, and biological factors external to a person, and all the related factors impacting behaviours. It encompasses the assessment and control of those environmental factors that can potentially affect health. It is targeted towards preventing disease and creating health-supportive environments. This definition excludes behaviour not related to environment, as well as behaviour related to the social and cultural environment, and genetics.
>
> (World Health Organization 2018)

In my view, given current knowledge on the interrelation and inter-connectedness between the physical environment and the social and cultural environment, this definition could usefully be reviewed and broadened in scope.

Core local authority environmental health functions in England include dealing with housing standards; food safety; health and safety; air pollution control; contaminated land; control of statutory nuisances such as noise, dust and odour; and in dealing with communicable diseases. Additional functions might include imported food control in port areas; licensing; food standards; statutory burials; health promotion; and enforcing 'smoke-free' legislation. Environmental Health Practitioners are one of very few public health occupational groups with a regulatory role and statutory powers, for example, being able to serve various notices, including for improvement, seizure, detention and prohibition and to take criminal prosecutions. Their wide remit has also led to them being referred to as the 'general practitioners of public health' (Cornell 1996: 74).

However, several policy areas have also impacted upon environmental health, particularly in terms of a diminution of the regulatory role as part of the 'Better Regulation' agenda, 'Red Tape Challenge', 'Focus on Enforcement' and other similar initiatives. Local government budgetary cuts have also impacted on the scope of services and have led to a retraction and focus on statutory functions which in turn impacts on the ability of practitioners to play a full role as public health professionals.

Academic commentators have criticised 'the government's ideological war on enforcement', raising concerns at the growing trend of under- rather than over-enforcement (James, Tombs et al. 2013: 49–50), and Day cites Professor Hugh Pennington as stating (food hygiene) 'inspections should not be regarded as a burden' (2011: 62). Nevertheless, this direction of travel has continued and presents a challenge to the environmental health profession as to how it defines itself for the next generation and how the regulatory role is funded and supported.

Looking at more positive developments, there have been recent calls for higher levels of taxation and regulation for health improvement (Triggle 2018), and the Local Government Association (2016) has produced a case study document supporting restrictions of hot takeaway premises around schools – a good example of how change can be made by working with other professional groups with overlapping interests

There is good reason to encourage innovation and growth of the environmental health remit beyond the specific limitations of enforceable legislation, and there is great scope for taking ownership of non-statutory activities within the broad area of environmental health. My former students and colleagues working in majority world countries are fully aware of this, as they take action to improve conditions in settings where the legislative framework may be dated or where resources for enforcement are lacking. An example in the UK may be where the legal framework is in place to enforce food hygiene and allergen controls, but opportunities to explore the causes of obesity or undernutrition are not included in the typical food safety role.

Environmental health and upstream interventions

The WHO has endorsed Acheson's 1988 definition of public health as 'the science and art of preventing disease, prolonging life and promoting health through organised efforts of society' (Jakab 2011: 4), and it recognises that one of the greatest public health challenges in Europe today is the 'unequal distribution of health and wealth'. This puts the issue of health inequalities centre stage for the public health professions, including the specialism of environmental health.

Marmot and Wilkinson (2006) describe the 'causes of the causes' of health inequalities as the 'social determinants of health', using the example of smoking contributing to many diseases. The social determinants in this case would not be cigarette smoking, but the reasons why people smoke. Marmot identifies the following as key determinants of health:

> … material circumstances, for example whether you live in a decent house with enough money to live healthily; social cohesion, for example whether you live in a safe neighbourhood without fear of crime; psychosocial factors, for example whether you smoke, eat healthily or take exercise; and biological factors, for example whether you have a history of particular illnesses in your family. In turn, these factors are influenced by social position, itself shaped by education, occupation, income, gender, ethnicity and race. All these influences are affected by the socio-political and cultural and social context in which they sit.
>
> (2010: 39)

The factors determining health are very well illustrated in Dahlgren and Whitehead's (1991) famous Main Determinants of Health model, and from this perspective it is clear that environmental health practitioners have a central role in the 'living and working conditions' domain (Figure 2.1).

The Main Determinants of Health

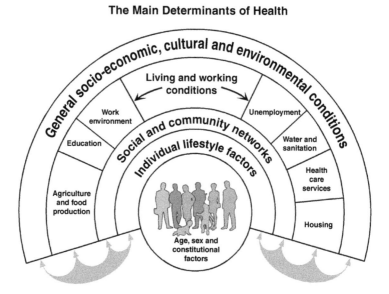

Source: Dahlgren and Whitehead, 1993

Figure 2.1 Dahlgren and Whitehead's Main Determinants of Health model illustrating the social determinants of health.

The idea of social determinants of health recognises that many important factors influencing health outcomes originate 'upstream' and therefore need to be addressed at that level, that is, dealing with social and economic structures rather than on healthcare interventions. Thus, policies to address the social determinants by their nature require a multifaceted approach across agencies and professional groups and are relevant to the role of public health policymakers. However, Bambra has noted previous policies and initiatives have focused too heavily on 'downstream' measures and notes that an upstream approach needs to be maintained (Bambra 2012).

The work of environmental health practitioners is by its nature upstream, based as it is on preventing ill health and accident in the home, workplace and elsewhere. A key example is action to ensure safe and energy-efficient private sector housing, thus helping to protect the health and safety of the most vulnerable members of society, keeping people well rather than dealing with the consequences of an adverse occurrence.

Building upon Dahlgren and Whitehead's model, Raworth (2017) produced the 'Doughnut Model', which in addition to environmental elements, such as food, water, housing and work, considers matters of social justice, equality and political voice. Importantly, the model also takes into account sustainability and highlights the need to live within the planet's boundaries, ensuring that we do not over- or under-consume resources and consume according to our physical and social needs. This model is very helpful in conceptualising the impacts of environmental activities across the broad social and environmental determinants of health, with work on matters such as air pollution control also being recognised as important factors (Figure 2.2).

There are many models and theories as to why health inequalities exist (these will be discussed further in Chapter 3). Addressing these factors has been described as an important objective across the life

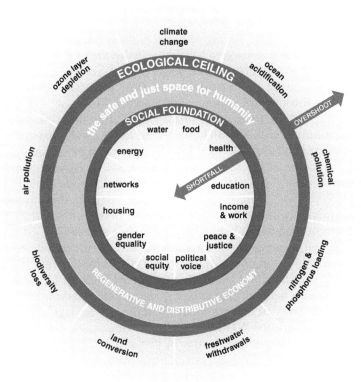

Figure 2.2 Raworth's 'Doughnut Model'.

course in the 'Marmot Review' as well as being a matter of social justice for the avoidance of unnecessary suffering (Marmot 2010). Health inequalities also have serious economic consequences with an estimated cost to the UK economy of £36 billion through a combination of lost taxes, healthcare costs and welfare payments.

In his groundbreaking review, Marmot identified key areas for prioritisation:

1   Giving every child the best start in life
2   Enabling all children, young people and adults to maximise their capabilities and have control over their lives
3   Creating fair employment and good work for all
4   Ensuring a healthy standard of living for all
5   Creating and developing sustainable places and communities
6   Strengthening the role and impact of ill-health prevention.

It is clear that every one of these priorities touches upon the environmental health remit, particularly if considered beyond narrow statutory constraints. Yet my research findings have shown that the potential for the profession to contribute in this area have been largely underestimated by public health policymakers, and the case has not been clearly made by practitioners or their professional body, the Chartered Institute of Environmental Health (CIEH).

In England, the Index of Multiple Deprivation describes relative deprivation and is used as an indicator for living conditions in different geographical areas. It takes into account a number of factors, including income, education, crime, health, housing, environment and unemployment. It is a useful tool for public health policymakers and practitioners and current evidence strongly suggests that mortality rates are highly linked to income (Dunnell, Blakemore et al. 2018).

Environmental health inequalities, whilst not well recognised in the UK, are well acknowledged at international level and are considered a serious matter of 'environmental justice' across the European region (World Health Organization Regional Office for Europe 2012: 16). Of particular importance are housing, injury and environment-related inequalities.

There is now an international commitment to tackling health inequalities, with the WHO stating 'Improving health for all and reducing health inequalities' as one of two strategic objectives set out in the Health 2020 European policy framework. This should serve to increase the policy focus on initiatives in the UK and bring opportunities and some leverage for environmental health practitioners to grasp the potential their roles offer.

Professional identities in environmental health

Given the changing role and title over the years of what is currently known as environmental health, and the fluctuations in central government support for public services, local government and the regulatory role, professional identities deserve some consideration. For example, what does it mean to be an environmental health practitioner in the 21st century? What is our relationship to the other public health professions? What is the status of the profession? And where should we be positioning ourselves in the coming decades in order to have the greatest impact on the health of the public we serve? This book aims to answer some of these questions and the themes are revisited in the conclusion; however, consideration of the environmental health identity in relation to tackling health inequalities is relevant here.

Several factors have been found to contribute to professional identity (of healthcare practitioners), including working environment, society, training, education and skills and registration to practice (Professional Standards Authority 2018). In my research, I found a combination of views around what it meant to be an environmental health practitioner; some of the most challenging issues were the extent to which the profession and duties are limited to the statutory role and of whether practitioners are strongest professionally as generalists or specialists. The interdisciplinary nature of environmental health also adds a layer of complexity around professional identity, which is an asset but also a vulnerability in that there is a lack of a 'home and body of knowledge' (Barratt, Couch et al. 2013) These issues continue to be debated and to influence how practitioners see themselves, their strengths and their weaknesses and how we train and support the new generation (Dhesi and Lynch 2016).

Looking at the wider more theoretical literature, Lipsky helpfully identifies and defines 'street-level bureaucrats' as 'public service workers who interact directly with citizens in the course of their jobs, and who have substantial discretion in the execution of their work' (Lipsky 1980: 3). Initially, I considered this rather an insulting label but have come to appreciate that the concept offers a very helpful perspective when considering the role and freedoms of environmental health practitioners to develop policy in addition to implementing it. This is important when considering the opportunities for practitioners on the ground to shape local government policy implementation around tackling the social determinants of health.

Moving to consider the types of issues front-line environmental health practitioners deal with, Day (2011) acknowledges the work of Schön when he notes that 'the firm high ground presents the problems that are immediately solvable through the application of well-understood theory and practice, but are relatively unimportant in the grand order of things, and the "swampy lowlands" which contain problems which are "messy and confusing" but are of far greater importance to society and the objectives of the profession'. This illustrates nicely some of the challenges facing the environmental health profession – do we focus our energies on technical issues with clear solutions; or do we tackle the 'swampy' issues such as health inequalities; or do we try to do both? In my view, we must embrace the latter option for the greatest opportunities to protect and promote the public's health.

References

Allen, P. (1991). "Environmental health officers." In *Health through Public Policy*. Ed. P. Draper. London, Green Print: 135–143.

Ashton, J. and H. Seymour (1988). *The New Public Health*. Buckingham, Open University Press.

Bambra, C. (2012). "Reducing health inequalities: new data suggest that the English strategy was partially successful." *Journal of Epidemiol Community Health* 66(7): 662.

Barratt, C., R. Couch, A. Page, S. Dhesi, and J. Stewart (2013). "An Introduction to Evidence Based Environmental Health." Retrieved from http://ukehrnet. wordpress.com/2013/09/11/research-briefing-1-introducing-evidence-based-eh/, UK Environmental Health Network (EHRNet).

Betts, G., Ed. (1993). *Local Government and Inequalities in Health*. Aldershot, Avebury.

Cornell, S. J. (1996). "Do environmental health officers practise public health?" *Public Health* 110(2): 73–75.

Dahlgren, G. and M. Whitehead (1993). *Tackling inequalities in health: what can we learn from what has been tried?* Working paper prepared for the King's Fund International Seminar on Tackling Inequalities in Health, September 1993, Ditchley Park, Oxfordshire, London, King's Fund, accessible in: Dahlgren, G. and M. Whitehead (2007). European strategies for tackling social inequities in health: Levelling up Part 2. Copenhagen: WHO Regional office for Europe: www.euro.who.int/_data/assets/pdf_file/0018/103824/E89384.pdf.

Day, C. (2011). "Environmental health – its practice and promotion." In *Clay's Handbook of Environmental Health*. Ed. S. Battersby. London, Routledge: 51–84.

Dhesi, S. and Z. Lynch (2016). "What next for environmental health?" *Perspectives in Public Health* 136(4): 225–230.

Dunnell, K., C. Blakemore, S. Haberman, K. McPherson, and J. Pattison (2018). *Life Expectancy: Is the Socioeconomic Gap Narrowing?* www.longevitypanel.co.uk/_files/LSP_Report.pdf.

Green, J. and N. Thorogood (1998). *Analysing Health Policy; A Sociological Approach*. London, Longman.

Griffiths, S. (2003). "Public health in the United Kingdom." In *Global Public Health: A New Era*. Ed. R. Beaglehole. Oxford, Oxford University Press: 54–68.

Hamlin, C. (2013). "Nuisances and community in mid-Victorian England: the attraction of inspection." *Social History* 38(3): 346–379.

Hatchett, W., S. Spear, J. Stewart, J. Stewart, A. Greenwell, and D. Clapham (2012). *The Stuff of Life. Public Health in Edwardian Britain*. London, CIEH.

House of Commons Select Committee on Health. (2001). Second Report House of Commons. https://publications.parliament.uk/pa/cm200001/cmselect/cmhealth/30/3008.htm.

Jakab, Z. (2011). *Your Health Is Your Wealth: A Policy Framework for a Healthier Ireland 2012–2020*. Dublin, World Health Organisation.

James, P., S. Tombs, and D. Whyte (2013). "An independent review of British health and safety regulation? From common sense to non-sense." *Policy Studies* 34(1): 36–52.

Lewis, J. (1986). *What Price Community Medicine?* Brighton, Wheatsheaf Books.

Lipsky, M. (1980). *Street-Level Bureaucracy: Dilemmas of the Individual in Public Service*. New York, Russell Sage Foundation.

Local Government Association. (2016). *Tipping the Scales. Case Studies on the Use of Planning Powers to Limit Hot Food Takeaways*. London.

MacGibbon, B. (1997). *Agendas for Change*. London, Chadwick House Group.

Marmot, M. (2010). *Fair Society, Healthy Lives: Strategic Review of Health Inequalities in England Post 2010*. London, UCL.

Marmot, M. and R. Wilkinson (2006). *Social Determinants of Health*. Oxford, Oxford University Press.

Professional Standards Authority. (2018). *The Regulator's Role in Professional Identity: Validator Not Creator*. London.

Raworth, K. (2017). "What on Earth is the Doughnut?...." *Exploring Doughnut Economics*. Retrieved from www.kateraworth.com/doughnut/.

Triggle, N. (2018). "Tax and regulate more to improve health." Retrieved from www.bbc.co.uk/news/health-44621038.

World Health Organization. (2018). "Environmental health." Retrieved from www.searo.who.int/topics/environmental_health/en/.

World Health Organization Regional Office for Europe. (2012). *Environmental Health Inequalities in Europe*. Copenhagen.

3 Tackling health inequalities

The causes of health inequalities

Health inequalities are complex and enduring and have frequently been called 'wicked problems' (Hunter, Marks et al. 2010: 158; Exworthy and Oliver 2012: 291), in that they are difficult to address and overcome or, more controversially, problems 'for which there may be no solution' (Allen and Rowse 2013: 21).

It is now widely accepted that there are links between mortality rates and age, gender, class and employment (Mitchell, Shaw et al. 2000) and that with some exceptions, poorer people are associated with shorter lives and poorer health than richer people (Benzeval, Judge et al. 1995; Davey Smith 2003). This effect, known as the 'health gradient', occurs between and within every social class or socio-economic group and sees the people at higher positions experiencing better health than people at lower positions (Marmot and Wilkinson 2006). It is also known that advantaged groups are also experiencing faster health gains than less advantaged groups (Graham 2009), and some predict that there could soon be rises in mortality rates for certain disadvantaged groups (Dorling 2013).

There is also a great deal of evidence to support the existence of health inequalities between social groups and in different geographical areas, linking health inequalities with place; for example, there is a North-South divide in England, with people in the more affluent South living longer, illustrated by the 9.2-year life expectancy difference for males in East Dorset and Blackpool (Office for National Statistics 2013). Others have found ethnicity to be a determinant of health and inequalities (Karlsen, Nazroo et al. 2002; Rao, Chandra et al. 2010).

In whatever way health inequalities are expressed, defined or measured, all the evidence represents a great deal of avoidable suffering and many lost years; indeed, it has been noted that 'between 1.3 and 2.5 million extra years of life could be gained by reducing health inequalities in England' (The Lancet Editorial 2010: 525). As Marmot says, 'Inequalities are a matter of life and death, health and sickness, wellbeing and misery' (Marmot 2010: 37), and this brings with it a moral imperative.

More recently, the WHO has stated that 'The term "health inequalities" refers to general differences in health. Many of these differences (particularly where they are linked to social variables or gender) represent "health inequities" because they are unfair, unjust and avoidable' (World Health Organization Regional Office for Europe 2012: 15). Unfortunately, to confuse matters, the terms equity and equality often appear to be used interchangeably in the literature. It is thus unsurprising that the term 'health inequalities' will mean different things to different people.

There are many models for understanding health inequality, and these are very helpfully summarised by Mel Bartley as cross-sectional, life course and macrosocial (2017). The life course approach was subscribed to by Marmot (2010) in the 'Fair Society Healthy Lives' strategic review of health inequalities and subsequently adopted by the then government. Davey Smith (2003) states that this explanation of health inequalities began with the work of Forsdahl and later Barker, who initially considered that childhood malnutrition led to higher rates of coronary heart disease in adulthood. Davy Smith goes on to state that they later came to the conclusion that more powerful than childhood conditions was the nutrition experienced in utero. This led to the concept that the nutrition and other conditions throughout life could affect health, which became known as the life course approach.

Other theories include the idea that the prolonged stress of a 'social-evaluative threat' creates a constant 'fight or flight' reaction, where cortisol is released, leading to physical effects including cardiovascular problems, obesity and psychological effects such as increased aggression (Wilkinson and Pickett 2010).

An alternative but partly linked theory proposed by Scott-Samuel (2011) is that health inequalities stem from societal power inequalities. These include the neo-liberal capitalist system, the lack of emotional literacy in leaders and the patriarchal religious system, which he says will prevent any progress being made in the current context, and (as I have described earlier) others agree that the neo-liberal system is widening inequalities (Coburn 2004). There are many other theories relating to specific groups such as women, ethnic minorities and people living in certain geographical areas. In measuring these (and the traditional class) factors, there has been criticism of the lack of information and routine recording of information required to measure health inequalities (Townsend, Davidson et al. 1988; Fulton 2010).

Unfortunately, some explanations can lead to 'victim blaming', for example, Pitts (1996) highlights the 'Just World Hypothesis', where it is believed that someone brings their own misfortune. She uses the stigma and blame attached to HIV/AIDS and diseases arising from smoking and obesity as examples of this, differentiating between 'innocent victim' and 'thoroughly deserving victim'. The Edwardian idea of the 'deserving' and 'undeserving' poor (Spear 2012) and the concept of there being a 'morality to poverty' has recently re-emerged in some media reports (Wynne-Jones 2013) along with the 'chav' stereotype of the working class (Jones 2011). Others have observed that the Coalition government used 'anti-welfare populism' promoting resentment and a view of the poor as 'other' to enable cuts to the welfare system to be made (Hoggett, Wilkinson et al. 2013), although welfare systems benefit wider society in the form of pensions, education, healthcare and the effects of redistribution of wealth (Hills 2015). Nathanson (2010: 274) nicely sums up issues of blame around inequalities:

> Inequalities attributed to sinful indulgence in wine and women are much less likely to interest penny-pinching public authorities than those attributed, for example, to the handle on the Broad Street pump.

The relevance of this phenomenon to the public health is evident in the potential impacts both on and of the decision-making of local elected members (and others) on the balance between individual responsibility and the role of society in tackling health inequalities, and their consequent prioritisation and commissioning decisions.

As we have seen, the causes of health inequalities are highly complex, and they remain the subject of some speculation and ongoing research. As such, they are not straightforward either to define or to address, and there are difficulties in evaluating the short- and medium-term effectiveness of interventions which may only be apparent in the long term. Bambra (2012: 662) cautions 'the importance of time lags when measuring the effects of interventions on health inequalities, especially multiple interventions that may result in a combined effect over time'. These lags can cause problems where funding is based on short-term outcomes and where the electoral system results in pressure to demonstrate policy impacts in one term.

Unsurprisingly, there are many suggestions as to what might work in tackling health inequalities. In the 'Fair Society Healthy Lives' review, Marmot suggests the six policy objectives listed in Chapter 2.

Interestingly, none of these priorities focus specifically on healthcare, and many of the Marmot priorities are in the domains of professional groups such as educators, welfare and benefit policymakers, environmental health practitioners and planners.

Nevertheless, there is significant support from scholars on the need to tackle poverty; for example, Mitchell and colleagues (2000) consider that the number of premature deaths in Britain would decline if there was full employment, a modest redistribution of wealth and an end to childhood poverty. There is a difference, however, between improving the economic circumstances of the poorest people and creating economic equality in a society. Bosma (2009) suggests that policymaking for equality may have more of an impact on general health and poverty reduction than health inequalities, citing genetic and cultural issues as also being important.

Understandings of health inequalities and prioritisation

My research has revealed that the Marmot objectives were popularly adopted as a framework by public health policymakers, but that some interviewees felt that this was more a matter of timing and an absence of alternatives rather than a deep commitment to the policy objectives compared to other possible frameworks. There was some concern (although this was a minority view) that Marmot objectives may lead to unrealistic expectations and might not be readily applicable at a practical level. There was also some tension between the priorities of different professional groups involved in policymaking and Marmot provided a framework which could be agreed to by a range of policymakers from different backgrounds.

In looking at enacting of policy in relation to Marmot, it is useful to start with case study site 3, which was very committed to the Marmot policy objectives and had set up an operational group of high-level individuals devoted to the implementation of the Marmot principles locally.

At case study site 1, the selecting of priorities for joint strategy was very much the work of the public health team, and this was disappointing to a healthcare representative who felt they should have been consulted on the adoption of the life course approach (as advocated by Marmot), but was nevertheless willing to implement the strategy in their own policies:

> ...and it just would have been helpful to say: do you want to take the life course approach, do you want to have focus on children and elderly? And then in fact, I think what they came up with was really good and it is things that we can easily pin health priorities

to but I just, I personally don't feel as a member of the public health policymaking group, that we would have particular owner-ship of either really, although I'm happy to pick it up and run with it and that's what we have to do, but I just think we could have shared in the understanding much more effectively....

(Public health policymaker ID17, site 1)

It can be seen that Marmot policy objectives have played a large role in influencing approaches to tackling health inequalities, particularly being seen as a useful starting framework for discussion. The influence of Marmot at a local level, where two policy objectives relate specifi-cally to children and young people, can be seen in the prioritisation of children as a population group in the developing strategies by inter-viewees of different backgrounds. A commitment to prevention and addressing the social determinants of health was in evidence during the majority of interviews, although observations at all case study sites noted a focus on healthcare and social care during many public health policymaking group meetings.

It appeared that there were two approaches to issue-based priori-tisation: focusing on specific population groups, such as children or vulnerable people, and focusing on health issues, such as smoking, drugs and alcohol, dementia or obesity. Sites generally adopted a mixture of both issue-based approaches, and there was little real support seen for geographical prioritisation other than in primary healthcare, where the provision and quality of care were sometimes referred to as issues.

In line with the Marmot objectives, there was a great deal of support for a focus on children from policymakers with a variety of backgrounds, elected members and officers:

...for me, the children's directorate has a tremendous role in the [public health policymaking group]. Now, one of the frustrations I had initially was it was all about adults and older people and so, I firmly, in my [health care organisation], have put resource and energy into getting the right people around the children's agenda, because, for me, that links very strongly with the preventative agenda and if we get that right, we often pick up lots of other things, dysfunctional family units, mental health issues, drug and alcohol problems, so, you know, it all, kind of, links together re-ally, but I feel quite strongly that we mustn't lose the children's agenda ... [it shouldn't be] playing second fiddle to anything, it should actually drive a lot of the other things.

(Public health policymaker ID5, site 3)

An environmental health manager described a local focus on education, children, older people and obesity, which whilst not being explicitly labelled as tackling health inequalities were likely to have an impact:

> ...that first meeting was quite driven towards education in children, which is fine and not an incorrect priority, but we need to be a bit wider than that. And health inequalities do play into that .... so, I think rather than saying our local [public health policymaking group] has picked out health inequalities as a key area, I don't think they have, but I think that, the thinking is actually we need to look at education in children, a little bit about older people as well, and obesity. Health inequalities are actually fundamental to those. So it's almost the other way around, we're not saying we haven't, but actually we're focusing on these areas and health inequalities is a fundamental part of them.
>
> (Environmental health manager ID47, site 18)

An interviewee with a public health role felt that alcohol, particularly in relation to young people, was the most pressing issue locally:

> Alcohol is our biggest challenge I would say. We're something like the [one of the] highest nationally for under 18 admissions for alcohol. Right up there as well for adults as well. Huge impact. Huge culture of drinking being the norm and not seen as a problem. So in terms of health priorities that's absolutely mine.
>
> (Public health policymaker ID26, site 4)

An elected member at the same site with both a health service and local authority background felt that raising expectations by focusing on education was important, with a message of individual empowerment:

> ...the underlying cause, in my view, not the expert's view, not Public Health's view, my personal view is it's around lack of expectations. Absolutely, so people don't strive education-wise, what's it all about? My Mum's never worked – my father's never worked, you know, my brother doesn't work, this is what's meant for me in life .... So there's a big, huge task of trying to empower people to say: No. I can do better. I'm going to choose a different pathway .... So you know, in many ways it does start with education then doesn't it?
>
> (Public health policymaker ID25, site 4)

A member with a public health role felt that there was a risk that their department could dominate, with other voices being unheard:

> I think there's a risk that it's going to be too public health focused. I mean I could fill the board agenda …. But we need to support those other agencies to say it's your board as well and you're not just here to listen to what's going on in public health, you're here to bring your partnerships in.
>
> (Public health policymaker ID26, site 4)

As we have seen, there was generally a focus on an issue-based approach to prioritisation rather than on geographical areas. There was no overt disagreement seen about this approach to prioritisation, although some interviewees did note that (healthcare organisation) representatives were often focused on their geographical areas rather than the 'bigger picture'. This was interesting, as there were many voices advocating many priorities, and it appeared that the issue-based approach facilitated an agreed strategic direction. The rationale was explained by a public health policymaking group member:

> Now, on a strategic basis, something like [area] quite clearly you've got more affluent people with loads more money who can drink loads more red wine and get liver disease down in the south. Then you go to [area] where you drink strong lager and smoke yourself to death or go and nick cars or whatever. So therefore people have a different perception of what they mean by inequalities and how that's presented … I've always had this belief … that actually if you identify an issue, say, alcohol, it is alcohol we're going to tackle and it doesn't matter where you live …. So let's look at the illness and let's tackle the illness. Don't do it on a geographical scale.
>
> (Public health policymaker ID21, site 1)

An environmental health manager in a very rural lower-tier authority felt it was important that local decisions were made on issue-based prioritisation, noting that child obesity was an issue in some areas of the county, but not in their district:

> …child obesity is not a big problem here, because we're a very old district … inequalities for us are around older people. The inequalities for us, is real, is very, very real, about access to services because … there is no rural transport.
>
> (Environmental health manager ID44, site 15)

Not all interviewees were so clear on what should be prioritised. One elected member expressed uncertainty in what should be done to tackle health inequalities:

> What more can the local authority do to help [other organisations] in driving down health inequalities? I mean we all know what they are, you know, we live 10 years shorter in [area] than we do in [area] and you know, teenage pregnancies, obesity, it's all worse in the North than it is in the South ... think we've got to see what we can do about [it], I'm not sure we actually know.
>
> (Public health policymaker ID9, site 2)

An environmental health manager felt that it was the quality of life rather than the length of life which should be the focus and priority in tackling health inequalities:

> So what we are doing is making people live longer, but we're making them live longer with illnesses and disabilities, and that is a difficulty for their life. So in terms of health inequality, our role, I feel, is, is to narrow the gap between illness and death ... if you die at ninety, but you act like a thirty year old, well then you've done your business. And to have a massive terminal drop, so you know, you've got fitness, fitness, fitness – dmp! – as opposed to that gradual decline into old age, and that is, from my point of view, is what health inequality is about.
>
> (Environmental health manager ID37, site 10)

A policymaker representing the voluntary sector was concerned about the impact of external policy decisions, feeling that the welfare system changes would make tackling health inequalities much more difficult:

> ...so actually we're just going to make health inequalities worse with welfare benefit reform, with all of the things that people are facing .... We're about to enter into a whole new era I think of not that far from Dickensian England. And that's the worrying thing, because actually you're just compounding issues for people, aren't you?
>
> (Public health policymaker ID28, site 4)

An environmental health practitioner took an even wider view, saying they believed that health inequalities were caused by much larger issues than the public health policymaking group could act on locally:

> ...what I believe will have the most fundamental effect on it obviously is reducing poverty and reducing the gradient difference between being poor and being rich in this country .... So unfortunately our economic philosophy doesn't really work with that. So being a capitalist society ... you get the worst gradient. So it's really to do with economics, war, housing, education, all these big things ...
>
> (Environmental health practitioner ID45, site 16)

There have been several critiques of the Marmot review and its recommendations, although these appear to have come from academics rather than practitioners. Several commentators have criticised the vagueness of recommendations, particularly at the national level (Whitehead and Popay 2010), and others have raised concerns at the focus on individual empowerment to 'take control of one's life', which is in contrast to upstream measures promoted elsewhere in the review and 'is by no means a guarantee of good health' (Nathanson and Hopper 2010: 1238). Whitehead and Popay were unimpressed by the focus on action at a local level and also that the role of political power and other wider factors were overlooked (Subramanyam, Kawachi et al. 2010). Pickett and Dorling (2010: 1231–1233) also felt that the failures to promote wider changes in UK society and 'to deal with the need to reduce inequality by focusing on the top end of the social hierarchy, as well as at the bottom' were significant omissions, and they ask, 'Why did the Marmot review not make hard-hitting recommendations to reduce the harm created by great differences in rank and status?' Concerns have also been raised that the review did not address ethnic factors in health inequalities (Fulton 2010), and the economists Chandra and Vogl (2010) provide a detailed critique of the evidence used to support some of the claims of causality in the review. Finally, others hold the view that a downstream focus on healthcare can have a great impact in tackling health inequalities (Nathanson and Hopper 2010), particularly by targeting the most disadvantaged during early childhood (Canning and Bowser 2010).

The British Academy asked nine academics to suggest local authority action to reduce health inequalities. Their suggestions were introducing a living wage, reducing speed limits, focusing on early childhood, tackling worklessness, focusing on mental health and capacity, using further and adult education, looking at ethnicity, developing older age-friendly environments and basing decisions on good evidence and evaluation (Pickett, Melhuish et al. 2014). The King's Fund also produced a resource pack for local authority public health prioritisation (Buck and Gregory 2013).

Returning to my research findings, there were also mixed feelings on whether the enactment of policies in practice would make any difference to health inequalities locally, as a support officer candidly said:

> Addressing health inequalities is bloody difficult. My personal view is I kind of question whether specific actions even make any difference to health inequalities, when you're looking at such a grand scale. You know, half a million people ... the kind of macro-economics, it's like a drop in the ocean basically. You try and do all this kind of community stuff and get people to go to their screenings, and then unemployment doubles and all the work is washed away within six months.
>
> (Public health policymaker support officer ID14, site 1)

Most other interviewees were more positive about potential impacts; however, many examples given focused on very limited or tightly defined issues. Marmot was also found to have featured heavily in the local policymaking process, and this is seen in the following comment from a support officer, who explained the value of the principles as a framework at a site where commitment to Marmot was proudly promoted:

> ...all Marmot did was help us to set priorities, it's just a framework, you can choose any other framework if you want, they're all, kind of, saying the same thing. We're very clear, children, years 0–5 very important, preventative agenda and getting that right, mental health, huge issue in [area], hidden communities, massive issue in [area] and then the long term conditions, cardio respiratory problems and linking into that, diabetes, smoking, obesity and all the rest of it, so you can feed out from them and, so, the point is, actually, I don't think we're going to argue over those priority areas, which is where I think Marmot took us to ...
>
> (Public health policymaker support officer ID5, site 3)

A policymaker representing a healthcare organisation at the same site agreed that Marmot had provided a useful framework for agreement at an early stage:

> I think, Marmot resonates with me, as a general practitioner, because it looks at all the life stages and that's fine, but it's only

telling me what I knew already, so it's good to be reassured by that, but I'm not hung up about whether it's Marmot, or any other framework they use, I want to use a framework that everyone agrees on, initially, and can stick to and says, fine, let's go forward with this, it doesn't give us the answers, it just highlights the issues and where we ought to start.

(Public health policymaker ID5, site 3)

Marmot was also subscribed to by many of the environmental health practitioners and managers interviewed:

To me, health inequalities is about having different health outcomes as a result of where you are born, or who you are born to, basically, and it's about unfairness and having your life cut short just because your parents weren't middle class or above and there is a gradient, so it's not just that poor people die earlier, it's that if the poorest people die the earliest and the middle poorest die the middle of that – so the social gradient that Marmot identified really, yeah, I really subscribe to that, definitely.

(Environmental health practitioner ID45, site 16)

An environmental health manager explained the reasons for the focus on Marmot in local policies and strategies, namely that it provided a point of focus at the right time:

I think it also came out at the same time and it was the flavour of the moment and it was a good way to go, it gave everybody a direction and something to hang on to...

(Environmental health manager ID48, site 19)

An environmental health manager at a different site added that the lack of other available guidance had led to their focus on Marmot when writing local policies and strategies:

...at the time, this was written before the public outcomes framework came into being, so the only thing we'd got to base it on really was Marmot...

(Environmental health manager ID4, site 3)

...each of the local authority reps have got a lead for one of the outcome themes of Marmot and ... we're trying to join it all up at the moment ... trying to join the dots, cause there's lots of dots so you've got a health protection strategy, health inequalities strategy, there's about 5 or 6 that's all thematic. So what we're trying to do is link those to the Marmot outcomes and actually match that to the lifecycle, so that you know, you get born in a healthy way, you die with dignity ...

(Environmental health manager ID3, site 3)

In contrast to the enthusiasm seen at this site, an environmental health practitioner with a national role explained the concerns about Marmot being seen as a 'panacea':

...these panaceas really worry me, I wish they were true. I wish somebody would give us the panacea, and we just go out and do it, but there's been plenty of opportunities in the past and they haven't worked yet.

(Environmental health practitioner
with national role ID33)

They went on to talk about their concerns about how the Marmot principles could be adopted at a practical level to make a difference and voiced their disappointment at the failure of central government to adopt the policy objective relating to poverty to 'ensure a healthy standard of living for all' (Marmot 2010: 116):

... and then Marmot comes along, with all that reinforcement about reading at bedtime and stuff and yeah, I'm sure it all counts. But again, if I'm just sitting there in my scruffy flat, with not enough to eat and up to my neck in debt and being abused, you know, by society and partners and everything am I really in a frame of mind to be told the best thing I can do is read to my kids or is that the practical level at which we need to start and say, actually we can't do anything about your housing at the moment, alright, and you are going to be poor for the foreseeable future, but these are things you can do and I don't know which way we go on all that ... but we'd better sort it out because it's no good trying to do everything and failing at so much, we need some successes .... Marmot's important, yes. The bit of Marmot I'm most interested in, the bit the government hasn't signed up to was poverty.

(Environmental health practitioner
with national role ID33)

We can see that whilst there are a range of opinions expressed as to what health inequalities are and what should be done about them, the majority of research participants felt able to endorse Marmots policy objectives, although perhaps with different emphasis, and this provided common ground to work on.

Planning actions to tackle health inequalities

Prior to Marmot's review, the Black Report (Townsend, Davidson et al. 1988) specifically listed improving working conditions and housing as necessary to tackle health inequalities. Evans and Killoran (2000: 136) agree that 'health strategies and programmes need to address such "upstream" determinants of health as poverty, unemployment and poor housing if the health of the worst off in society is to be improved'. The (new) Labour government, elected in 1997, accepted that there were many social determinants of health and focused policies on addressing a broad range of these (Uberoi, Coutts et al. 2009); however, the results cannot realistically be measured in the short to medium term (Sassi 2005).

My research found some inconsistencies in what people said or 'espouse' about health inequalities and what they actually proposed to do or 'enact' in practice. There were both similarities and differences in the understandings and priorities espoused by individuals and subsequently enacted by policymakers as priorities in their strategies.

As would be expected, there are many suggestions as to what might work in tackling health inequalities. For example, Mitchell and colleagues (2000) consider that the number of premature deaths in Britain would decline if the economic factors such as full employment, redistribution and ending childhood poverty were addressed. The idea of poverty reduction as a means to tackling health inequality seems to have widespread academic support (Benzeval, Judge et al. 1995), although this has not received governmental support. Margaret Whitehead, cited by Benzeval et al. (1995), suggests that policies can reduce health inequalities at four levels through the following:

- Strengthening individuals
- Strengthening communities
- Improving access to essential facilities and services
- Encouraging macroeconomic and cultural change

Researchers have discussed many other factors. For example, some research indicates that in more equal societies, there is less ill health and fewer social problems (Wilkinson and Pickett 2010), and others agree that action on social and economic justice in society is needed to address public health issues (Labonte, Frank et al. 2008). Others argue that apparent equality could be masking other inequalities such as those between men and women (Bartley 2017). Fulton (2010) also notes that although many governments have published strategies aimed at tackling health inequalities, the majority have focused on socio-economic factors, omitting to consider ethnicity as a significant factor.

It is evident that there is no agreed approach to tackling the causes of health inequalities. Some say that economic redistribution (Sassi 2005) would address the issue, whilst others argue that education (Blaxter cited by Bartley [2004]) or direct health interventions (Canning and Bowser 2010) are the answer and proponents of the life course approach stress the importance of action at different life stages (Marmot 2010). Nevertheless, the causes of health inequalities are complex and multifactorial, and only a minority can be addressed by the health service (Asthana and Halliday 2006b). The Environmental Health Commission (MacGibbon 1997) particularly noted the need for 'bottom-up' action with the strong involvement locally of members of the public.

In developing social and economic policies to tackle inequalities, it is important to note that options for improving population health in general may do nothing for closing the gap in health inequalities. Sassi (2005) points out that the Labour government controversially held the view that increasing overall population health would reduce health inequalities, as those most in need would be the greatest beneficiaries. He contrasts this approach with that of the previous Conservative administration, which relied on an economic recovery based on a 'trickle-down' strategy. A review paper looking at the success of government reviews in reducing health inequalities found that 'reforming left-leaning governments are more committed to long-term monitoring of inequalities, even if the results are not always politically comfortable' (Howden-Chapman 2010: 1242).

As we have seen, the reasons suggested for health inequalities are complex, and this is recognised by the National Institute for Health and Care Excellence (NICE) guidelines, which add that social and material circumstances can affect the abilities of individuals to change or modify their behaviour (National Institute for Health and Clinical Excellence 2007). Connected to this is a need to look more closely at the 'causes of the causes' including the reasons why certain behaviours are practiced. There is also a concern that the current enthusiasm for 'nudge' could widen health inequalities, as different members of society will be able to respond in different ways to health messages (Standing 2011a).

The concept of nudge is built around offering a 'choice architecture', where individuals are encouraged, often covertly, to make 'good' decisions whilst still having the option of selecting 'bad' ones (Thaler and Sunstein 2009). Proponents of this approach, also referred to as 'behavioural insight', argue that this 'libertarian paternalism' approach is a low-cost way of improving population health whilst maintaining individual liberties and therefore acceptable to the political right, where 'nannying' is unpalatable. However, the claim of preserving individual liberties is arguably not strictly true when the intention is to manipulate behaviour, and others highlight the role of powerful industries in talking down the 'nanny state' and preventing necessary action on public health issues (Wiley, Berman et al. 2013).

Thaler and Sunstein (2009) note that the approach is also being used to promote health-damaging behaviours, citing existing examples of nudge used to promote driving instead of walking and the consumption of unhealthy foods and excessive alcohol (Bonell, McKee et al. 2011; Marteu, Ogilvie et al. 2011). Examples given by the Cabinet Office of case studies 'applying behavioural insight to health' are the introduction of the National Food Hygiene Rating Scheme, which provides inspection information to consumers; a mentoring scheme for likely teenage mothers to spend time with toddlers; changing 'norms' of drinking by publicising low average consumption to university students; and a smoking cessation trial with the pharmacist Boots (Cabinet Office Behavioural Insights Team 2010; Hawkes 2011).

Opponents of the approach argue that it is unethical to try to change behaviour without the consent of the individuals involved; that it is coercive and rewards 'bad' behaviour (Oliver and Brown 2011); and that it changes motivation from acting for the reason of 'doing the right thing' to acting because a (monetary or other) reward is offered. Additionally, there are concerns around equity, where 'nudges' or 'conditionality' are targeted only at certain groups of people (for example, those on low incomes) rather than applying across society. Tied to this is the notion that some people are more 'deserving' than others (Standing 2011b), and here we have a link to the 'victim blaming' discussed earlier. Bonell et al. (2011: 11) argue that

> ...the government had misrepresented nudging as being in opposition to their use of regulation and legislation to promote health, and that this misrepresentation serves to obscure the government's failure to propose realistic actions to address the upstream socioeconomic and environmental determinants of disease.

Others point out that the evidence of nudge for positive behaviour change is weak (Marteu, Ogilvie et al. 2011); nevertheless, it remains a powerful concept.

The observation that health improvements cannot be made solely by medical means or by relying on an individual's sense of personal responsibility is not a new discovery. MacGibbon (1997) notes that McKeown found in the 1970s that improved mortality rates (the small-pox vaccination aside) from 1840 onwards were due to family size limitations, food supplies and environmental improvements made possible through general economic growth. Whilst this view is well recognised, it is challenged by Szreter (1988), who contests economic growth as being beneficial and emphasises the role of local government in securing improvements. Clearly, neither argument supports the role of medicine as the main driver in improving population health, and it seems to me that good local governance and economic growth should not be mutually exclusive.

The work of Marks et al. (2010) identified a tension between the collective and the individual in focus groups discussing the new public health arrangements. In treating society or a group of people as a unit, the behavioural approach can be contrasted with the 'collective protection' approach mandated in legislation and guidance in the field of occupational health and safety, a key area of environmental health practice. To illustrate, the majority of occupational health and safety regulations now explicitly require that collective measures pro-tecting all individuals take precedence over individual controls. This hierarchical approach recognises that reliance on human behaviour is untenable; indeed, investigations have found 'human factors' to be the major causes of several very serious incidents: for example, Piper Alpha, Chernobyl, Bhopal, King's Cross and Zeebrugge (Health and Safety Executive 2005).

Additional examples of where a collective approach has successfully been taken to protect public health in the UK include the introduction of the Clean Air Acts, the requiring of the provision of potable wa-ter and, most recently, the 'smoke free' legislation. Other examples of effective societal approaches are the criminalisation of drink-driving, the introduction of annual vehicle safety tests and the requirement to wear a seatbelt. All demonstrate that legislation can effectively change lifestyle behaviour (Kopelman 2011). Such approaches are also useful where the necessary action cannot be taken by those who are affected, for example, with food hygiene standards in commercial premises or providing basic protection for homeless people. All these are situations where changes have been mandated for the collective good of society, although clearly this approach is not appropriate in all situations, and a balance must be made with individual liberty. Arguments for the use of legislation in public health can be explained as follows:

> Legislation can appear to be a simple and powerful tool, and the evidence suggests that introducing legislation, in conjunction with other interventions, can be effective at individual, community and population levels.
>
> (National Institute for Health and
> Clinical Excellence 2007: 8)

The Nuffield Council on Bioethics' (2007) 'intervention ladder' describes a stepped approach to interventions, with legislation being seen as a 'last resort' when the other steps have been exhausted. However, an argument can be made for initial action involving the restriction or elimination of choice where imminent risks to public health exist (Figure 3.1).

Assertions against the use of regulation in public health interventions can be summed up by the following quote:

> Strong-armed regulation is not the answer to rebalancing our diets, changing our desire to drink too much alcohol on a Friday night, or making our lives more active.
>
> (Cabinet Office Behavioural Insights Team 2010: 6)

Whilst initially, and as discussed earlier, it seems that these approaches could be complimentary, Asthana and Halliday (2006a) contribute a topical observation, pointing out that right-wing policies for addressing

Eliminate choice
Restrict choice
Guide choice by disincentives
Guide choice by incentives
Guide choice by changing the default policy
Enable choice
Provide information
Do nothing

Figure 3.1 Nuffield Council on Bioethics intervention ladder.

health inequalities tend to focus on the choices of individuals, whereas left wing policies see poorer health as the outcome of the material circumstances of certain groups. Politics and public health are invariably intertwined and are discussed in more depth later in this book.

Both nudge and enforcement or regulation have their proponents, and it has been argued both that the approaches are mutually exclusive and that they are not (Bonell, McKee et al. 2011). The original definition of nudge excluded legislation (Marteu, Ogilvie et al. 2011), but legislation was used in examples listed by the originators of the idea in their book (Thaler and Sunstein 2009). The background literature on nudge and political attitudes to enforcement and regulation are important for this book, which focuses on the role of environmental health, which to date has been primarily a regulatory public health occupation.

References

Allen, S. and J. Rowse (2013). "Health and well being boards – developing transformational relationships." *Journal of Integrated Care* 21(1): 19–25.

Asthana, S. and J. Halliday (2006a). "Developing an evidence base for policies and interventions to address health inequalities: the analysis of 'Public Health Regimes'." *The Milbank Quarterly* 84(3): 577–603.

Asthana, S. and J. Halliday (2006b). *What Works in Tackling Health Inequalities? Pathways, Policies and Practice through the Lifecourse.* Bristol, Policy Press.

Bambra, C. (2012). "Reducing health inequalities: new data suggest that the English strategy was partially successful." *Journal of Epidemiol Community Health* 66(7): 662.

Bartley, M. (2017). *Health Inequality: An Introduction to Theories, Concepts and Methods.* Cambridge, Polity Press.

Benzeval, M., K. Judge, and M. Whitehead, Eds. (1995). *Tackling Inequalities in Health: An Agenda for Action.* London, Kings Fund.

Bonell, C., M. McKee, A. Fletcher, A. Haines, and P. Wilkinson (2011). "Nudge smudge: UK Government misrepresents 'nudge'." *The Lancet* 377(9784): 2158–2159.

Bonell, C., M. McKee, A. Fletcher, P. Wilkinson, and A. Haines (2011). "One nudge forward, two steps back." *BMJ.* 342 (7791): 241–242

Bosma, H. (2009). "A critical reflection on the role of social democracy in reducing socioeconomic inequalities in health: A commentary on Sekine, Chandola, Martikainen, Marmot and Kagamimori." *Social Science & Medicine* 69(10): 1426–1428.

Buck, D. and S. Gregory (2013). *Improving the Public's Health.* London, The King's Fund.

Cabinet Office Behavioural Insights Team. (2010). *Applying Behavioural Insight to Health.* C. Office. London, Cabinet Office Behavioural Insights Team.

Canning, D. and D. Bowser (2010). "Investing in health to improve the wellbeing of the disadvantaged: Reversing the argument of *Fair Society Healthy Lives* (The Marmot Review)." *Social Science and Medicine* 71: 1223–1226.

Chandra, A. and T. S. Vogl (2010). "Rising up with shoe leather? A comment on *Fair Society, Healthy Lives* (The Marmot Review)." *Social Science & Medicine* 71: 1227–1230.

Coburn, D. (2004). "Beyond the income inequality hypothesis: class, neoliberalism, and health inequalities." *Social Science and Medicine* 58: 41–56.

Davey Smith, G., Ed. (2003). *Health Inequalities: Lifecourse Approaches*. Bristol, The Policy Press

Dorling, D. (2013). *Think Piece. In Place of Fear: Narrowing Health Inequalities*. Class, Centre for Labour and Social Studies. London, Class.

Evans, D. and A. Killoran (2000). "Tackling health inequalities through partnership working: learning from a realistic evaluation." *Critical Public Health* 10(2): 125–140.

Exworthy, M. and A. Oliver (2012). "Evidence and health inequalities: the Black, Acheson and Marmot reports." In *Shaping Health Policy. Case Study Methods and Analysis*. Eds. M. Exworthy, S. Peckham, M. Powell, and A. Hann. Bristol, Policy Press: 291–310.

Fulton, R. (2010). "Ethnic monitoring: is health equality possible without it?" *Race Equality Foundation* Better Health Briefing (21) https://raceequalityfoundation.org.uk/wp-content/uploads/2018/03/health-brief21.pdf.

Graham, H. (2009). "Health inequalities, social determinants and public health policy." *Policy and Politics* 37(4): 463–479.

Hawkes, N. (2011). "Finding the techniques to nudge the population to better health." *BMJ* 342 (7791): 241–242.

Health and Safety Executive. (2005). "Inspectors toolkit: human factors in major hazards, Appendix 1." Retrieved 25.01.11, 2011, from www.hse.gov.uk/humanfactors/topics/toolkit.pdf.

Hills, J. (2015). *Good Times Bad Times. The Welfare Myth of Them and Us*. Bristol, Policy Press.

Hoggett, P., H. Wilkinson, and P. Beedell (2013). "Fairness and the politics of resentment." *Journal of Social Policy* 42(3): 567–585.

Howden-Chapman, P. (2010). "Evidence-based politics: How successful have government reviews been as policy instruments to reduce health inequalities in England?" *Social Science and Medicine* 71: 1240–1243.

Hunter, D. J., L. Marks, and K. E. Smith (2010). *The Public Health System in England*. Bristol, Policy Press.

Jones, O. (2011). *Chavs. The Demonisation of the Working Class*. London, Verso.

Karlsen, S., J. Y. Nazroo, and R. Stephenson (2002). "Ethnicity, environment and health: putting ethnic inequalities in health in their place." *Social Science and Medicine* 55(9): 1647–1661.

Kopelman, P. (2011). "Debate: tackling obesity – to 'nudge' or to 'shove'?" *Public Money and Management* 31(4): 236–238.

Labonte, R., J. Frank, and E. Di Ruggiero (2008). "Introduction." In *Critical Perspectives in Public Health*. Eds. J. Green and R. Labonte. London, Routledge: 14–23.

MacGibbon, B. (1997). *Agendas for Change*. London, Chadwick House Group.

Marks, L., S. Cave, and D. Hunter (2010). "Public health governance: views of key stakeholders." *Public Health* 124: 55–59.

Marmot, M. (2010). *Fair Society, Healthy Lives: Strategic Review of Health Inequalities in England Post 2010*. London, UCL.

Marmot, M. and R. Wilkinson, Eds. (2006). *Social Determinants of Health*. Oxford, Oxford University Press.

Marteu, T. M., D. Ogilvie, M. Roland, M. Suhrcke, and M. P. Kelly (2011). "Judging nudging: can nudging improve population health?" *BMJ* 342(7791): 263–265.

Mitchell, R., M. Shaw, and D. Dorling (2000). *Inequalities in Life and Death. What if Britain Were More Equal?* Bristol, Policy Press.

Nathanson, C. A. (2010). "Who owns health inequalities?" *The Lancet* 375(9711): 274–275.

Nathanson, C. and K. Hopper (2010). "The Marmot Review – social revolution by stealth." *Social Science & Medicine* 71(7): 1237–1239.

National Institute for Health and Clinical Excellence (2007). *Behaviour Change at Population, Community and Individual Levels*. London, NICE.

Nuffield Council on Bioethics. (2007). *Public Health: Ethical Issues*. London, Nuffield Council on Bioethics.

Office for National Statistics. (2013). "Statistical bulletin: Life expectancy at birth and at age 65 for local areas in England and Wales, 2009–11." Retrieved 09.08.13, 2013, from www.ons.gov.uk/ons/rel/subnational-health4/life-expectancy-at-birth-and-at-age-65-by-local-areas-in-england-and-wales/2009-11/stb.html.

Oliver, A. and L. D. Brown (2011). "Incentivizing professionals and patients: a consideration in the context of the United Kingdom and the United States." *Journal of Health Politics, Policy and Law* 36(1): 59–87.

Pickett, K. and D. Dorling (2010). "Against the organization of misery? The Marmot Review of health inequalities." *Social Science & Medicine* 71(7): 1231–1233.

Pickett, K., E. Melhuish, D. Dorling, C. Bambara, K. McKenzie, T. Chandola, A. Jenkins, J. Nazroo, H. Kendig, C. Phillipson, and A. Maynard (2014). *'If you could do one thing'. Nine Local Actions to Reduce Health Inequalities*. London, British Academy.

Pitts, M. (1996). *The Psychology of Preventative Health*. London, Routledge.

Rao, J. N., J. Chandra, and P. Jennings (2010). "Ethnicity, health and health inequalities." *Ethnicity and Inequalities in Health and Social Care* 3(2): 4–5.

Sassi, F. (2005). "Tacking health inequalities. Health, poverty and social exclusion." In *A More Equal Society?* Eds. H. J and K. Stewart. Bristol, Policy Press: 69.

Scott-Samuel, A. (2011). "Further evidence that effective interventions on health inequalities must tackle the root causes." *2011;342:d3460.*

Spear, S. (2012). "The workhouse." In *The Stuff of Life. Public Health in Edwardian Britain.* Ed. William Hatchett and Stuart Spear London, CIEH: 109–121.

Standing, G. (2011a). "Behavioural conditionality: why the nudges must be stopped – an opinion piece." *Journal of Poverty and Social Justice* 19(1): 27–38.

Standing, G. (2011b). *The Precariat: The New Dangerous Class.* New York, London, Bloomsbury Academic.

Subramanyam, M. A., I. Kawachi, and S. V. Subramanian (2010). "Reactions to fair society, healthy lives (The Marmot Review)." *Social Science & Medicine* 71(7): 1221–1222.

Szreter, S. (1988). "The importance of social intervention in Britain's mortality decline c.1850–1914: a re-interpretation of the role of public health." *Social History of Medicine* 1(1): 1–38.

Thaler, R. H. and C. R. Sunstein (2009). *Nudge: Improving Decisions about Health, Wealth and Happiness.* London, Penguin Books.

The Lancet Editorial. (2010). "Health equity – an election manifesto?" *The Lancet* 375(9714): 525.

Townsend, P., N. Davidson, and M. Whitehead (1988). *Inequalities in Heath: The Black Report and the Health Divide.* Harmondsworth, Penguin.

Uberoi, V., A. Coutts, I. McLean, and D. Halpern, Eds. (2009). *Options for a New Britain.* Basingstoke, Palgrave Macmillan.

Whitehead, M. and J. Popay (2010). "Swimming upstream? Taking action on the social determinants of health inequalities." *Social Science and Medicine* 71(7): 1234–1236.

Wiley, L. F., M. L. Berman, and D. Blanke (2013). "Who's your nanny? Choice, paternalism and public health in the age of personal responsibility." *Journal of Law, Medicine and Ethics* 41: 88–91.

Wilkinson, R. G. and K. Pickett (2010). *The Spirit Level: Why Equality Is Better for Everyone.* London, Penguin.

World Health Organization Regional Office for Europe. (2012). *Environmental Health Inequalities in Europe.* Copenhagen, World Health Organization Regional Office for Europe.

Wynne-Jones, R. (2013). "Deserving vs undeserving." Retrieved 09.08.13, 2013, from www.jrf.org.uk/reporting-poverty/journalists-experiences/deserving-undeserving.

4 Public health policymaking

The public health systems and structures in England

As I have described, the role of local government in public health has been subject to structural and functional change over a number of years. Whilst the literature is extensive and cannot be fully discussed here, an understanding of how authorities are structured and operate is crucial in appreciating the differences between the health service and other organisations and in understanding the findings of the research on which this book is based.

The organisation of local government in England is complex and can be confusing. In the majority of cities and some counties, authorities are described as 'unitary': that is, all functions are carried out by one body. In other areas, there are two tiers, with some functions, such as social services, education, trading standards and highways, sitting at the upper tier, whilst other functions, such as environmental health, building control and planning, sit at the lower level. However, these terms can be misleading, as upper-tier authorities do not have any jurisdiction over district and borough councils, and indeed the latter prefer to be called 'district councils' (Gray 2013). All are independent organisations, although they do work closely where beneficial, for example, in emergency planning and protecting food standards.

Local authorities are 'creatures of statute'; that is, they exist to carry out specific functions prescribed in law and are 'a provider of services to a local community and an instrument of democratic self-government, not a mere agent of the state' (Redcliffe-Maud and Wood 1974: 10). They are controlled by locally elected members (councillors), usually one for each ward or parish, and just as in central government, party politics play a significant role, a development which has increased since the 1970s (Wilson and Game 2006). This democratic element, particularly the ability to make decisions affecting communities at a local level, is important, but it can lead to tensions when this is in conflict with nationally set targets or strategic priorities.

Elected councillors may be independent or stand as members of a political party or other interest group. Typically, the turnout for local elections is low (the lowest in Western Europe), at times as low as around 30–40% (Bogdanor 2011), and there is a general 'indifference and disinterest' in local politics (Pratchett 2004). This apathy also relates to elected members and has been described by Michael Heseltine, cited by Byrne (1994): 'it's getting harder to attract people to serve on councils. Not just the people of the necessary calibre – it's often difficult to attract anyone at all'. Pratchett also lists four reasons why 'local politics does not work': public indifference; elected members not being representative of the communities they serve; poor links with partners and the community; and their paternalistic approach (Pratchett 2004). All these factors could potentially play a role in the operation and quality of decision-making of local government bodies with responsibilities for public health.

Councillors make key decisions on budgets and strategy and are guided by officers, who are responsible for day-to-day management (Bassett 1995). This distinction between roles has been described as useful but simplistic, and other theories or models suggest that officers hold the balance of power or that decision-making is balanced between elected members and officers (Wilson and Game 2006) or that there is a 'dynamic dependency' between them even where the vision or agenda is not shared (Gains 2004). Whichever model is subscribed to, it is clear that the relationships and power balance between officers and elected members can be nuanced and complex (Gains, John et al. 2008). This is very important given the unusual membership of the public health policymaking bodies researched for this book, where councillors and officers have equal voting rights and necessarily need to switch to their former roles for other duties.

In March 2013, the Communities and Local Government Committee published its report on the role of local authorities in health, which acknowledged their role in prevention and tackling the social determinants of health and noted that work across all services is needed (House of Commons Select Committee on Health, Communities and Local Government Committee 2013). It is clear that there are many functions in both tiers which can have an impact on the social determinants of health. The Improvement and Development Agency (I&DeA) has carried out a substantial piece of work entitled 'The social determinants of health and the role of Local Government' (Campbell 2010) which looks at many of the factors in my research.

Of particular interest is the chapter by Dorling in which he talks about 'place shaping', which proposes an alternative view of local government that moves away from focusing on the statutory delivery of individual services towards 'a unit of government, responsible for the wellbeing of a community and a place, and independent of, whilst also being connected to, the wider system of government' (2010). This alternative view fits well with the idea of the public health policymaking group as a forum for the health and well-being of a geographical area across services; organisations and recent work on place shaping, including Health Impact Assessment in the North-East, found that the approach bought strategic advantages in relation to understanding the wider determinants of health locally.

Following the major restructure of 1974, various efforts have been made to encourage joint working between healthcare services and local authorities towards common goals (Evans and Killoran 2000; Smith, Bambara et al. 2009), with several policies promoting partnership working between these organisations (Coleman, Checkland et al. 2014). Joint working was mandated in the Health Act 1999, which requires that National Health Service (NHS) bodies and local authorities cooperate to improve the health and welfare of the population. However, partnership working is not straightforward, as geographical boundaries have not necessarily matched, and practices and language can be quite different, as are governance arrangements, duties and responsibilities. Evans and Killoran (2000) found that whilst strategies may need to talk about 'joined up thinking for joined up problems', there is 'a difficult reality of securing integrated action on the ground'. Others add that the historic division between health and social care functions has led to 'a series of practical barriers to effective joint working which continue to frustrate service users and staff and to consume significant management time' (Glasby, Dickinson et al. 2010), and Coleman et al. (2014) have also found that there needs to be commitment from all organisations and individuals within health and social care partnerships for effective working.

Given the policy emphasis in recent years, it is natural and easy to assume that partnership working is a 'good thing', that it is beneficial and yields positive results. The evidence is less convincing: a systematic review of the impact of organisational partnerships on health outcomes found that 'there is little evidence of the direct health effects of public health partnerships' (Smith, Bambara et al. 2009). To complicate matters, the concept of 'partnership' means different things to different people and organisations, and as such, initiatives can be difficult to evaluate (Glendinning 2002).

Public health policymakers are by their nature inter-organisational and inter-professional. Glendinning (2002) points out that different professional groups will have different approaches, for example, in the selection of services considered appropriate to involve for a given outcome; for example, Betts found that health services take an 'individualistic approach', whereas local authorities favour 'collective action' (1993). A House of Commons report stated that it was hoped the recent structural changes would facilitate a move from a medical model to a social model of health, focusing on prevention (House of Commons Select Committee on Health, Communities and Local Government Committee 2013), so the concepts are important for public health policymakers and environmental health practitioners alike.

The World Health Organization (World Health Organization 2013) has acknowledged (in relation to disability) that there are limitations in both the social and medical models and has proposed the use of the 'biopsychosocial' model, which combines the personal and environmental factors, as an alternative. Organisations such as the UK Public Health Association have been pushing for public health to move away from the medical model towards the social model (House of Commons Health Committee 2011a). Evans and Killoran (2000) found that whilst strategies focus on joint working, it is difficult to achieve in practice; others add that the historic division between health and social care functions has led to 'a series of practical barriers to effective joint working which continue to frustrate service users and staff and to consume significant management time' (Glasby, Dickinson et al. 2010). Angela Mawle, chief executive of the UK Public Health Association, has drawn attention to the significant cultural difference in terms of training and elected member involvement (House of Commons Health Committee 2011a).

Staite and Miller add that in addition to cultural differences, there are also significant differences between professional groups involved in public health policymaking:

> The differences form icebergs – some are above the surface, but most lie below, unacknowledged, poorly understood and a hazard to effective partnerships. These include differences in roles, language and experience as well as the differences between those who work within the framework of local democracy and those whose political masters are in Whitehall.
>
> (Staite and Miller 2011)

Glendinning (2002) found influencing factors in partnership development and outcomes included the maturity of relationships and past experiences and encounters. This observation is important as new structures are often populated by individuals who have worked together previously in former initiatives.

Murphy points out that public health policymaking groups have built on the foundations of previous initiatives, such as Total Place and Local Area Agreements, that had similar objectives (Murphy 2013), which tells us there has been a great deal of research on the problems associated with partnership working between social care and the NHS. There has not been the same level of empirical research on partnership working for health between the NHS and other local authority departments or functions or other health partnerships, and to my knowledge, this is the first major research project focusing on the role of environmental health in public health policymaking.

The policymaking process

Given the broad themes covered by this research, an overarching conceptual framework offering an understanding of the policy context is helpful. Professor Stephen Harrison was a member of my supervisory team, and at an early stage in my PhD I attended the Teddy Chester Lecture given by him entitled 'Reorganising the English NHS 1974–2011: from design to doodle?' (Harrison 2011). The lecture described the different approaches to health policymaking from the major restructure in 1974 until what was then the present day. It built upon earlier work with Wood (1999), describing a change in policy detail from 'blueprint to bright idea' and 'manipulated emergence'.

The original 'manipulated emergence' concept noted that different administrative approaches had been taken for various health restructures. Starting with the reorganisation in 1974 (which was discussed in Chapter 1), Harrison and Wood note that a prolonged period of consultation and planning took place with extremely detailed guidance given on the expected structures and functions. They call this approach a 'blueprint' and argue that since then

> there has been a shift away from the presentation of a blueprint as the intended endpoint of reorganisation, and its replacement by the 'bright idea': a rather nonspecific vision of how to proceed. Second the role and timing of advice and consultation has changed from a situation where expert advice significantly shaped the content of the blueprint to one in which the expert contribution lay

in the translation by incentivised local actors of the bright idea into specific organisational arrangements which accord with the philosophy behind the original idea; we term this 'manipulated emergence'.

(Harrison and Wood 1999: 752)

Harrison and Wood go on to define what a 'bright idea' is, defining four elements: the development of policy in secret; providing limited details of the policy; allowing for later policy development; and implementation by incentivised volunteers. They were also clear in their view that the move from blueprint to bright idea cannot be directly linked to party politics; this is supported by others commenting on the 'pragmatic localism' of New Labour: '... it is a radically different sort of politics and policy making process where it appears that the ideology of political ideas has taken a back seat to delivering successful policy on the ground' (Coaffee and Headlam 2008: 1589).

Harrison's 'Design to doodle?' (2011) provides a useful conceptual framework for understanding the findings of this research. The idea that different levels of detail and prescription had been given by different central government administrations has stayed with me, and I have come to the view that the distinct lack of prescription and guidance offered by central government policymakers on the development of public health policymaking groups and the continued rise of the localism agenda, coupled with overt political values, provided a natural update to the spectrum concept proposed by Harrison.

The policy development and implementation for public health policymaking groups were carried out by local sites which were designated as 'early implementers'. Harrison and Wood (1999) comment on the nature of these local actor 'volunteers', noting that they gain from their association with a successful project and avoid the negative outcomes of not participating. The findings from my research indicate that there was an enthusiasm for involvement, with one case study site in particular putting great emphasis on being seen as a national leader in their development. The engagement of local actors led in most areas to their establishment well in advance of the passing of the legislation for the new policymaking structures to start working.

In my view, all four elements of Harrison's Bright Idea framework are met by the process of introducing public health policymaking groups. To illustrate, Murphy points out that there was no green paper on the proposals and 'precious little forewarning of the proposed extent of the reforms from either the Conservative or Liberal Democrat election manifestos or from the coalition agreement' (Murphy 2013:

250); I have described previously the system of volunteer 'early implementers' and the lack of central government guidance available.

I argue that the blueprint for the introduction of public health policymakers was also 'low', given that there was very little guidance available during the development stage. I am also taking the design to doodle spectrum one step further by linking the doodle or bright idea with the localism approach to their development seen during the research period. It appears to me that this new type of localism is the next step in the design to doodle spectrum, the difference being that of the inclusion of acknowledged political values, where the concept of decentralisation and localism was actively promoted by the coalition government, in particular with the passing of the Localism Act in 2011, introducing a 'general power of competence' for local authorities (although this is coupled with a limiting 'right to challenge'). Lowndes and Pratchett (2012: 22) have also noted the role of political values in a range of policies: '... the Coalition's reforms do show traces of an ideological commitment to localism and a new understanding of local self-government; there is an ideological agenda which has the potential to deliver a radically different form of local governance'.

The lack of clarity, particularly around expectations in relation to tackling health inequalities, led public health policymakers to search for evidence and guidance to support their strategic plans, and in some areas, they fell back on the templates of previous policies, strategies and arrangements.

For example, some context sites showed a lesser commitment to tackling health inequalities than the case study sites. In contrast to the majority of other sites, an environmental health manager at a context site explained that the existing strategies did not include priorities relating to the social determinants of health, but that this was based on previous initiatives and likely to change as they were reviewed:

> ...when you go back to the Joint Strategic Needs Assessment, those wider determinants aren't really in there, it's very much around the legacy of what was the local area agreement and the [area] Strategic Partnership and the priorities that were there got carried over and the strategy, you know, everybody will admit, was put together in a hurry really, so that the board had something to work to and could launch and that was it, but they've also recognised that in the next 12 months, we do need to refresh that ...
>
> (Environmental health manager ID35, site 8)

However, an environmental health practitioner at another authority also described how health inequalities were being treated as low priority:

> ...they've seen the word 'inequalities' and given it to our Social Inclusion Team to deal with and they've missed off the health, which obviously would be us, so it's been given, the Health Inequalities Plan has been given to a fairly junior member of the Inequalities Team to write. I don't think it's seen as particularly important ...
>
> (Environmental health practitioner ID45, site 16)

An environmental health manager (ID39, site 11) described the observations on differences in understanding and approach between healthcare and local authority colleagues with reference to Marmot. They explained that the medical approach would be to look at the issue or problem, consider the services available to deal with that problem and then set targets based upon the available resources. They went on to say that the local authority approach would also be to start with the issue or problem but would then look at how it might be solved, and finally they would put what was needed in place. It was their view that the latter approach was liberating and fitted with the Marmot philosophy, whereas the former did not.

There were clearly practical decisions to be made by different members of the public health policymaking group in balancing their different priorities and understandings whilst respecting those of others. This is well described by a public health policymaker:

> I'm not saying that there's a common sense of priority because ... the need to tackle the social determinants will be at different heights in the in-tray of different people [for example]... a general practitioner (GP) is predisposed to treat the symptoms rather than the underlying causes but the very high quality of GP leadership that we're enjoying through the CCGs are much better than any GP leadership I've seen in [area] historically, so I'm very pleased.
>
> (Public health policymaker ID7, site 3)

An environmental health manager at the same site described the concern that strategies tackling the social determinants must be accompanied by action plans for implementation, but that this approach was not appreciated by health colleagues, who were focusing purely on action plans for health services.

A public health policymaker support officer at the same site explained the work that had been done to overcome differences in understanding to ensure that the local authority was playing a full role in the new system, describing a shift in their practices:

> ...this morning, our chief executive asked me to have a look at some hospital performance data around people having too many follow up appointments in hospital and the amount of money that that is spending unnecessarily and, I think, previously, we would have approached that and said, 'well, it's an interesting area, but shouldn't we ask the hospital to give members an update on that', whereas, now it's more 'actually, [name], I want you to scrutinise that, come up with some issues that you think we might be able to get under, so that we're a bit more informed when we're asking the question'.
> (Public health policymaker support officer ID30, site 4)

In contrast, an environmental health manager explained that large projects on health inequalities in recent years had led to a common understanding in their area that social determinants of health were crucial, whilst recognising the differences in primary care provision demonstrating the role of local history:

> So I think everybody's got a pretty good handle on what health inequalities are and they don't like them and I think there's general understanding that it's not just about services ... people now have decided that half of the life expectancy gap is because of smoking trends and probably 25% of the life expectancy gap is down to other things that people do and bugger all is down to the quality of the doctor, although we do have good doctors gravitating to posh areas and bad doctors end up in the poorer areas.
> (Environmental health manager ID40, site 11)

There was often a lack of clarity about what strategic priorities would actually mean in practice and how they would be measured:

> ... What that means in practice, we haven't got to that yet ... and the health and wellbeing strategy has got to address how that's going to work really; what's generic, what's universal, what's targeted, and how are we going to know if it makes a difference?'
> (Public health policymaker support officer and
> environmental health manager ID8, site 2)

In two case study sites, there was a noticeable difference between the discussion of public health policymakers, as seen during observations, which were generally focused on healthcare and social care, and the content of the Joint Health and Wellbeing Strategy and other documents, which were produced by the public health teams and included a focus on the social determinants of health. This was explained by the support officer at one of those sites:

> ...although we've got Public Health leading this, there is recognition that the Health and Wellbeing Strategy is not a Public Health Strategy. It's a strategy for health and wellbeing and really the key determinants around health and wellbeing are jobs, housing – not public health. So I want to make sure that we've got slightly more of that in there. Although I have to say that we have had a bit of a disconnect between our Health and Wellbeing Strategy development and what the views of the board are, because I don't think the Board has been quite strong enough to sort of dictate exactly what it is it wants from the strategy.
>
> (Public health policymaker support officer
> ID6, site 3; my emphasis)

This disconnect could perhaps be a result of the pressure to produce significant strategic documents, whilst public health policymaking groups were very much at the development stage. The approach of the lead person drafting the Joint Health and Wellbeing Strategy appears to be important, as seen in some dissatisfaction from other groups external to site 1 to very aspirational targets in the Joint Health and Wellbeing Strategy relating to the social determinants of health, as a healthcare organisation representative of a public health policymaking group explained:

> ...we had a meeting with our partnership group in [area] where we discussed the strategy ... I don't know if it is to do with politics with a small p or what really, but people were not happy to talk about what they call 'motherhood and apple pie', targets around things like eradicating poverty or anything like that, they didn't want anything seen as so kind of impossible to achieve and you know, and so there's actually quite a lot of criticism of the strategy ... They were really quite, quite rude about it being too full of things that noone is ever going to achieve and just too aspirational and impractical.
>
> (Public health policymaker ID17, site 1)

In terms of the impacts and opportunities for the environmental health profession, the bright idea approach to public health policymaking does leave space for influencing the agenda; however, a coherent and compelling case is needed to stand out from the other groups vying for space (and funds).

Politics in policymaking

The health implications of recession and austerity policies have received attention in recent literature, with particular concerns raised around the effects on health, health services and health inequalities (Pearce 2013; Stuckler and Basu 2013; Wood 2013). It has been noted that there are both direct and indirect effects of austerity policies on health; direct effects are those on health spending, whereas indirect effects are those on social determinants of health, such as 'increasing unemployment, poverty and homelessness and other socio-economic risk factors, while cutting effective social protection programmes that mitigate their risks to health' (Reeves, Basu et al. 2013: 4).

Researchers from the Liverpool Public Health Observatory have identified several factors which they say separate the current economic downturn from previous recessions. These include falls in benefits (both unemployment and in-work) and earnings and the subsequent decline in living standards; new unemployment and worklessness; and changes in the nature of work, including loss of job security and employment rights, for example, in the growing 'gig economy'. They go on to say that the health effects of these manifest in stress, frustration-aggression (increasing violence and substance misuse) and actions to manage reduced incomes resulting in 'time poverty' limiting health-protecting activities (Winters, McAteer et al. 2012: 10). Others have highlighted the likely long- and short-term health effects of the recession and austerity policies in London. Again, these include the effects of reduced incomes (including from welfare reforms) and higher unemployment; they also predict increased suicides and perhaps homicides and increased domestic violence; an increase in the number of people with poor mental health; raise concerns around infectious disease outcomes, particularly for tuberculosis and HIV; and highlight issues around the health effects of poor housing and affordability (UCL Institute of Health Equity 2012). Both studies anticipate that the economic downturn will increase health inequalities, and this prediction is supported by others who have noted the negative effects of recession and austerity policies on health (Barr, Taylor-Robinson et al. 2012; Stuckler and Basu 2013; Wood 2013) and in particular of the global economic downturn on suicide rates (Chang, Stuckler et al. 2013). Others argue that the health effects are more nuanced and that, overall, there may be no effect (Pearce 2013).

There are also some limited positive health outcomes predicted, such as a decrease in road traffic fatalities as people reduce private car use (UCL Institute of Health Equity 2012).

There is a body of literature on the links between public health, political values and conditions (Stewart 2005; Mackenbach and McKee 2013; Pega, Kawachi et al. 2013), including, for example, Bambra, who cites Navarro's findings that administration by political parties with redistributive philosophies 'tended to have better health outcomes than those with more neo-liberal governments' (2011: 746). This view was endorsed by Mooney, who went as far as entitling the introduction to his book 'Neoliberalism Kills' (2012: 3), and Pearce also argues that the UK Conservative-led coalition government had used the financial crisis to suggest a 'crisis of big government' and exploited the circumstances as a rationale for extending 'neoliberal ideologies' (2013: 2030). Policies of austerity have continued to the time of writing. In addition, a report by NHS Health Scotland commented on the health effects of neo-liberal policies:

> The impacts of recession (and the policy responses to the recession) may impact differentially across the population (e.g. by gender, income group, social class, disability). It has been found that countries which pursue active labour market policies and provide improved social and welfare protection have populations with better health than those which do not, and those which pursue neo-liberal policies (i.e. reduced market regulation, increased privatisation and decreased universality of welfare provision) tend to see health inequalities widen.
>
> (McCartney, Myers et al. 2013: 9)

Pearce's (2013) comment on neo-liberalism in the UK can be directly related to the argument for the introduction of the legislation introducing the policymaking bodies on which my research is based, where much was made of the need for health reorganisation to cope with the spiralling cost of the NHS (Wood 2013). Although Hunter (2013) states that 'it has never been clear what the problem was to which the changes were presented as the solution', he goes on to comment on why the central government pushed through such an unpopular piece of legislation:

> Why the government should risk so much political capital by pressing ahead in such circumstances remains a puzzle. Unless, that is, one seeks to understand the political drivers behind the proposals. It is their ideological nature, and alignment with the government agenda committed to reducing the size of the state as an employer

in order to create private sector jobs, which may hold the clue to the government's dogged persistence to see its changes through.

(Hunter 2013: 12)

Others agreed that the government did not make it clear what the need or purpose for the changes were (Timmins 2012). The essence of arguments around neo-liberalism and poorer health outcomes centre on issues of power, social justice, societal and monetary inequality and of individual responsibility against that of society as a whole. It is evident that the possibilities for any local government structure in mitigating the health impacts of an economic downturn and the central government adherence to a neoliberal approach and policy of austerity will necessarily be limited.

Localism was a key part of the coalition government's agenda. In essence it means that decision-making should be at a local rather than a central level; it is about decentralisation. Nick Clegg, then the deputy prime minister, described it thus:

> Of course, the Liberal Democrats and Conservatives use different language to explain decentralisation and to fight its cause. The prime minister has coined the phrase 'Big Society' whilst the Liberal democrats tend to talk about 'Community Politics', or simply just 'Liberalism'. But whatever words we use, we are clear in our ambition to decentralise and disperse power in our society ....
>
> (HM Government 2010)

A further concern with the rise of the localism agenda is that local authorities are taking on additional duties at a time when they are experiencing severe funding pressures (House of Commons Health Committee 2011b). Clearly, this would affect their ability to respond effectively to the public health challenges in their local areas; indeed, Staite and Miller noted that large funding cuts 'will have the greatest impact on the most deprived areas where health inequalities present the greatest challenge' (2011: 2).

The political element is a feature of local government service provision. McCarthy (1996) says that environmental health programmes are linked to the social and political systems of the communities in which they are carried out, and this is also true of other local government functions, because local authorities are led by elected members who are directly accountable to the local community via elections. One of the reasons often given for the relocation of public health to local authorities was to restore the 'democratic deficit' of the NHS, in making decision makers accountable directly to the public. The NHS Confederation argues that since the secretary of state is responsible for the NHS, there is no existing deficit at a national level to be remedied (2011). As I have described, a consequence of giving elected members responsibility for decision-making is that these decisions can become politicised. A further consequence is that local decisions will vary in different areas. This is summed up neatly by David Hunter in his evidence to the Health Select Committee:

> Don't forget that this agenda is all about localism. Local authorities are different. That is the whole point about local government. They will vary in how they want to hold their Director Public Health to account, but that is the price of localism. You are either for it or against it, but if you buy it, you have to buy what goes with it, which is variation and difference.
>
> (House of Commons Health Committee 2011b)

Glasby et al., when discussing the idea of transferring all public health functions to local authorities, were of the opinion that this would increase interest in and turnout for local elections but that elected members 'may need considerable support and development to take on this new role' (2010: 256); Weiss (1999) also highlights the difficult balance and tensions between democratic and expert decision-making. These observations indicate that the issues raised about the role of elected members within the new system are important. The enhanced role for elected members and associated local politics could perhaps lead to a resurgence of one or both of the opposite approaches of the 'conviction politics' of Margaret Thatcher and the commitment to 'evidence-based policy' of New Labour described by Cookson, who is also of the view that the correct use of evidence-based policymaking may 'enhance open democracy and improve policy outcomes' (2005: 119).

On health and political values, Wilkinson points out (with reference to academics) that

> health inequality has always attracted the attention of people interested in social justice. But, at the same time, we have always shrunk from the inherently political nature of what it implies. Rudolph Virchow reminded us that 'medicine is politics and social medicine is politics writ large'...
>
> (2006: 1229)

Virchow, a cell biologist who later became a politician, made these comments in 1848, and the issue of how involved public health practitioners and academics should be in politics remains an area of discussion and debate today (Mackenbach 2009). A good example is that of Bambra (2014), who responded to criticism from the right-wing press to a paper she co-authored on the significant adverse health effects of the Thatcher-era policies. It is clear that researching the contentious issues of health and politics, as this project has touched upon, is far from straightforward and may have unforeseen implications.

It is clear that my research took place in a policy context of lo-calism as an espoused political value, and with the exception of a short list of statutory public health policymaking group members and the very open content of the legislation, there has been little attempt at prescribing local functions and structures. In drawing from the results of my research, it appears that the wide range of structures, substructures, the level of local involvement of environmental health and priorities are a direct result of the localism agenda which follows the doodle approach introduced by Harrison's spectrum. This brings with it both opportunities and threats for the environmental health profession.

References

Bambra, C. (2011). "Health inequalities and welfare state regimes: theoretical insights on a public health 'puzzle'." *Journal of Epidemiology and Community Health* 65: 740–745.

Bambra, C. (2014). "Thatcherism's lethal legacy and the politics of reporting research." Retrieved 14.02.14.

Barr, B., D. Taylor-Robinson, A. Scott-Samuel, M. McKee, and D. Stuckler (2012). "Suicides associated with the 2008–10 economic recession in England: time trend analysis." *British Medical Journal* 345(e5142).

Bassett, W. H., Ed. (1995). *Clay's Handbook of Environmental Health*. London, Chapman and Hall.

Betts, G., Ed. (1993). *Local Government and Inequalities in Health*. Aldershot, Avebury.

Bogdanor, V. (2011). *English Local Elections 5th May 2011*. Report and Analysis. Foreword.

Byrne, T. (1994). *Local Government in Britain*. Harmondsworth, Penguin.

Campbell, F. (2010). *The Social Determinants of Health and the Role of Local Government*. London, I&DeA.

Chang, S.-S., D. Stuckler, P. Yip, and D. Gunnell (2013). "Impact of 2008 global economic crisis on suicide: time trend study in 54 countries." *British Medical Journal* 347(f5239).

Coaffee, J. and N. Headlam (2008). "Pragmatic localism uncovered: the search for locally contingent solutions to national reform agendas." *Geoforum* 39(4): 1585–1599.

Coleman, A., K. Checkland, L. Warwick-Giles, and S. Peckham (2014). "Changing the local public health system in England: Early evidence from two qualitative studies of Clinical Commissioning Groups." Retrieved from www.prucomm.ac.uk/resources/our-publications/.

Cookson, R. (2005). "Evidence-based policy making in health care: what it is and what it isn't." *Journal of Health Services Research and Policy* 10(2): 118–121.

Dorling, D. (2010). "Using the concept of 'place' to understand and reduce health inequalities." In *The Social Determinants of Health and the Role of Local Government.* Ed. F. Campbell. London, Improvement and Development Agency: 16–25.

Evans, D. and A. Killoran (2000). "Tackling health inequalities through partnership working: learning from a realistic evaluation." *Critical Public Health* 10(2): 125–140.

Gains, F. (2004). "The local bureaucrat: a block to reform or a key to unlocking change?" In *British Local Government into the 21st Century.* Eds. G. Stoker and D. Wilson. Basingstoke, Palgrave Macmillan: 91–104.

Gains, F., P. John, and G. Stoker (2008). "When do bureaucrats prefer strong political principals? Institutional reform and bureaucratic preferences in English local government." *The British Journal of Politics & International Relations* 10(4): 649–665.

Glasby, J., H. Dickinson, and J. Smith (2010). "Creating NHS local: the relationship between English local government and the National Health Service." *Social Policy and Administration* 44(3): 244–264.

Glendinning, C. (2002). "Partnerships between health and social services: developing a framework for evaluation." *Policy and Politics* 30(1): 115–127.

Gray, I. (2013). *Personal Communication.* S. Dhesi.

Harrison, S. (2011). "Reorganising the English NHS 1974–2011: from design to doodle?" *The Teddy Chester Lecture.* University of Manchester. Version 2.

Harrison, S. and B. Wood (1999). "Designing Health Service Organisation in the UK, 1968–1998: From blueprint to bright idea and 'manipulated emergence'." *Public Administration* 77(4): 751–768.

HM Government (2010). *Decentralisation and the Localism Bill: An Essential Guide.* London, HM Government.

House of Commons Health Committee (2011a). *Corrected Transcript of Oral Evidence, Tuesday 7 June 2011. H. C. House of Commons.* London, House of Commons.

House of Commons Health Committee (2011b). *Corrected Transcript of Oral Evidence, Tuesday 17 May 2011. H. C. P. Health.* London, House of Commons.

House of Commons Select Committee on Health, Communities and Local Government Committee (2013). *The Role of Local Authorities in Health Issues. Eighth Report of Session 2012–13.* London, The Stationery Office.

Hunter, D. J. (2013). "Safe in our hands? Austerity and the health system." In *Health in Austerity*. Ed. C. Wood. London, Demos.

Lowndes, V. and L. Pratchett (2012). "Local governance under the coalition government: austerity, localism and the 'Big Society'." *Local Government Studies* 38(1): 21–40.

Mackenbach, J. (2009). "Politics is nothing but medicine at a larger scale: reflections on public health's biggest idea." *Journal of Epidemiology and Community Health* 63: 181–184.

Mackenbach, J. and M. McKee (2013). "Social-democratic government and health policy in Europe: a quantitative analysis." *International Journal of Health Services* 43(3): 389–413.

McCarthy, A. (1996). "Protecting the public health – the role of environmental health." *Public Health* 110(2): 77–80.

McCartney, G., F. Myers, M. Taulbut, W. MacDonald, M. Robinson, S. Scott, R. Mitchell, D. Millard, E. Tod, E. Curnock, S. Katikireddi, and N. Craig (2013). *Making a Bad Situation Worse? The Impact of Welfare Reform and the Economic Recession on Health and Health Inequalities in Scotland (Baseline Report)*. Edinburgh, NHS Health Scotland.

Mooney, G. (2012). *The Health of Nations. Towards a New Political Economy.* London, Zed Books.

Murphy, P. (2013). "Public Health and Health and Wellbeing Boards; antecedents, theory and development." *Perspectives in Public Health* 133(5): 248–253.

NHS Confederation (2011). "Where next for NHS reform?" A discussion paper. N. Confederation. London, NHS Confederation.

Pearce, J. (2013). "Financial crisis, austerity policies, and geographical inequalities in health." *Environment and Planning A* 45(9): 2030–2045.

Pega, F., I. Kawachi, K. Rasanathan, and O. Lundberg (2013). "Politics, policies and population health: a commentary on Mackenbach, Hu and Looman (2013)." *Social Science & Medicine* 93: 176–179.

Pratchett, L. (2004). "Institutions, politics and people: Making local politics work". In *British Local Government into the 21st Century*. Eds. G. Stoker and D. Wilson. Basingstoke, Palgrave Macmillan: 213–229.

Redcliffe-Maud, L. and B. Wood (1974). *English Local Government Reformed.* London, Oxford University Press.

Reeves, A., S. Basu, M. McKee, M. Marmot, and D. Stuckler (2013). "Austere or not? UK coalition government budgets and health inequalities." *Journal of the Royal Society of Medicine.* 106(11): 432–436

Smith, K. E., C. Bambara, K. E. Joyce, N. Perkins, D. J. Hunter, and E. A. Blenkinsopp (2009). "Partners in health? A systematic review of the impact of organizational partnerships on public health outcomes in England between 1997 and 2008." *Journal of Public Health* 31(2): 210–221.

Staite, C. and R. Miller (2011). "Health and Wellbeing Boards: developing a successful partnership." *I. o. L. G. S. University of Birmingham, Health Services Management Centre.* Birmingham, University of Birmingham.

Stewart, J. (2005). "A review of UK housing policy: Ideology and public health." *Public Health* 119: 525–534.

Stuckler, D. and S. Basu (2013). *The Body Economic. Why Austerity Kills.* London, Allen Lane, Penguin Books.

Timmins, N. (2012). *Never Again? The Story of the Health and Social Care Act 2012.* London, Institute for Government and the King's Fund.

UCL Institute of Health Equity (2012). *The Impact of the Economic Downturn and Policy Changes on Health Inequalities in London.* London, UCL.

Weiss, C. H. (1999). "The Interface between evaluation and public policy." *Evaluation* 5(4): 468–486.

Wilkinson, R. (2006). "Politics and health inequalities." *The Lancet* 368(9543): 1229–1230.

Wilson, D. and C. Game (2006). *Local Government in the United Kingdom.* Basingstoke, Palgrave Macmillan.

Winters, L., S. McAteer, and A. Scott-Samuel (2012). "Assessing the impact of the economic downturn on health and wellbeing." *Observatory Report Series No. 88.* Liverpool, Liverpool Public Health Observatory, University of Liverpool.

Wood, C., Ed. (2013). *Health in Austerity.* London, Demos.

World Health Organization (2013). *How to Use the ICF: A Practical Manual for Using the International Classification of Functioning, Disability and Health (ICF).* Exposure draft for comment Geneva, WHO.

5 Environmental health (in)visibility

Environmental health visibility

My research revealed that environmental health is doubly invisible, in that public health is culturally invisible, and within this sphere, environmental health is invisible. Practitioners and managers expressed difficulties in promoting their service to public health policymakers, their allied occupational groups and elected members, and a variety of reasons for this were proposed.

A major factor was the exclusion of environmental health from the nationally set statutory list of public health policymaking group members; this has been unhelpful in that health and social care issues have taken precedence, and environmental health is seen as one amongst many other groups vying for attention.

Public health has been described as being 'culturally invisible' to the outside world, as its achievements are eventually taken for granted and forgotten, and its impact is primarily based on what might happen – 'the drama of threat' and the occasional attention-grabbing crisis (Rayner and Lang 2012: 4–5), for example, a food poisoning outbreak or workplace fatality. My research suggests that environmental health is also invisible within the public health sphere, and it is likely that this is partly connected to the preventative role, where success means that adverse events do not happen:

> They're so good at what they do, you don't hear about them. You'd only hear about them if there were diseases all over the place and infections breaking out and premises being closed and all that.
>
> (Public health policymaker ID10, site 2)

As I have discussed earlier, environmental health is a local authority-based occupation, and local authorities may be structurally unitary or two-tiered, depending on the geographical area. My research results indicate that it struggles for recognition in both unitary and two-tiered areas, which is somewhat surprising given that environmental health is part of the same organisation as public health policymakers in unitary areas.

Some practitioners and managers in unitary authorities described the frustrations they felt in gaining recognition for the contribution of their services at an upstream, preventative level in local authority public health plans and strategies:

> I downloaded all the Health Inequality Plans I could find ... and they all do start with 'we have a huge problem with Mental Health, therefore we must sort out the services that people with mental health issues will have to contact'. But they don't actually look at what's caused the mental health issue and the problem in the first place. Is it because they are exposed to environmental factors that are destroying their mental health? And that's where Environmental Health comes in, and that's the bit that's not seen and not appreciated and included in these Health Inequality Plans. I haven't found one that includes anything to deal with the fact that Environmental Health deal with noise complaints and noise complaints have a massive impact on mental health ...
>
> (Environmental health practitioner ID45, site 16)

Environmental health practitioners and managers in two-tiered systems commonly felt that their role was unseen or ignored by public health policymaking group members and allied occupational groups based in the upper tier, although this could perhaps be a function of the structural arrangement rather than the overlooking of a particular profession:

> Well, some of the public health documents that have come out – I mean the way they view the local authority function – they're talking in terms of planning, in terms of culture, in terms of leisure – environmental health doesn't actually get a mention.
>
> (Environmental health practitioner ID38, site 10)

A manager at another site also felt that their service was largely unknown in the upper-tier authority:

> I would have thought at county level... they hardly know I exist ....
>
> (Environmental health manager ID36, site 9)

Other interviewees focused on the practical difficulties they had encountered in trying to gain recognition, both at a personal level and in relationships with medical colleagues, where there is often little common language or understanding:

> It's hard, at some of those meetings, you do feel a little bit overwhelmed by the background knowledge of some people coming; health and wellbeing strategy work that's been going on, the [public health needs assessment] work was very clinically orientated ... when I first sat on that group, and I thought to myself, this is an area we're so alien to ... with so many other people around the table, it's going to be quite difficult getting my voice heard.
>
> (Environmental health manager ID31, site 4)

Within local authorities, a common route for officers to keep elected members aware of developments in their service is to send reports for information to committee meetings. These differ from reports for action in that they are produced for awareness only and do not require decisions to be made. An environmental health manager in a district council described challenges in raising the profile of environmental health with elected members, as 'reports for information' were no longer being submitted and a restructure had removed the committee with specific responsibility for the service:

> The trend in the last few years, as you'll know, is that all the committees that we used to take information to, we used to have an environment health committee, ... [but] it's disappeared, so we don't have the information papers going to executive ... and so councillors generally don't hear about environmental health.
>
> (Environmental health manager ID 23, site 1; my emphasis)

During research interviews, I asked public health policymaking group members and support officers what they knew about environmental health; the majority of responses either revealed a very limited knowledge of the role or showed an awareness of few functions, primarily listing food hygiene as the main environmental health activity. The following comment is indicative of many responses:

> I: Can you tell me what you know about environmental health?
> R: Not a lot really, I mean, it's not really come to the board.
>
> (Public health policymaker ID5, site 3)

There were few interviewees who showed an understanding of even a small range of environmental health functions, although several expressed surprise at the extent of the role when they did find out about it (often as part of the research interview process), and this was the case within both two-tiered and unitary arrangements:

> I haven't had lots of opportunity to work with Environmental Health, but recently, I suppose, in the health agenda, that's when I have had the opportunity to find out a little bit more about their role and I've actually been quite surprised at their remit.
>
> (Public health policymaker support officer ID30, site 4)

In addition to having a very limited idea of the remit of environmental health, some interviewees greatly misunderstood the role, for example, mentioning street lighting and cutting bushes. A public health policymaking group member suggested the invisibility could be the result of a lack of understanding and appreciation of the environmental health role:

> I mean is it about people's understanding of what Environmental Health Officers do?
>
> (Public health policymaker ID11, site 2)

The feeling that members had very little understanding about the environmental health was supported by practitioners and managers, who felt it was misguided to assume that the role was obvious to others in the public health system:

> I think one of the mistakes that people make is that we sit back and go 'oh environmental health, everyone knows about us' and none of them do. They have no idea. No idea.
>
> (Environmental health manager ID37, site 10)

There were mixed responses regarding the understanding of the role by others working in public health, with the directors of public health generally better informed than their teams and colleagues on public health policymaking groups. An environmental health manager in a borough council described a positive response when public health colleagues were introduced to environmental health and understood the role:

> [The Public Health team] they've work shadowed, so they've been around, they spent a week going out with the environmental health

team, so they were, you know, they were blown away actually … they didn't realise just how much public health work we did.

(Environmental health manager ID41, site 12)

Others described a real sense of frustration in getting the message that environmental health is a public health specialism across to allied colleagues working in the area:

> I think people have just been exasperated, I've had a few people saying, oh, but we are Public Health, it's just we're Local Authority Public Health and it's, like, yes, I know, we need to keep repeating it to our new director of public health.
>
> (Public health policymaker support officer ID30, site 4)

This invisibility is strongly felt by environmental health practitioners and managers, who consider their service vital in protecting the public's health. However, this sense of importance does not appear to be shared by the majority of public health policymakers and allied professionals.

The questions arising from this evidence of invisibility within the public health community across the country are the following: does it matter? Does invisibility bring disadvantage? Or are there advantages to being invisible?

In my view, (in)visibility matters very much, particularly in an environment where funding is limited and multiple services are bidding for resources. An invisible environmental health service stripped back to its statutory functions will not be in a position to attract funding to support a full role in protecting the public's health. A secondary issue that follows is the ability of the profession to attract and retain bright and committed graduates when the scope of the role becomes narrow and the outcomes of the often challenging work is unrecognised, even by colleagues in the same field.

There were serious concerns expressed by several people about the future of environmental health being under threat, being doubly invisible and under-recognised in the new public health system, coupled with the negative effects of local authority spending cuts:

> And in better financial times Environmental Health Officers have been much more involved in terms of having much more health promotion type posts, but not being a statutory function, I think those tend to go when times get hard. So I don't know, and

> I suppose my sense is environmental health sort of retrenches to statutory functions when finances are tight.
>
> (Public health policymaker ID11, site 2)

Nevertheless, some interviewees expressed the view that the new public health policymaking arrangements offered opportunities as well as threats:

> My own view is, it's, if you don't embrace the opportunity, you are going to end up fighting with your existence in the not too distant future. So it's about, you know, we haven't got any choice and why would we want any choice actually, there's an opportunity here, there's an opportunity to make a real difference, let's grasp this.
>
> (Environmental health manager ID47, site 18)

Others agreed, feeling that the opportunities are there, but some effort on the part of environmental health is needed too:

> You know, do a bit of inward focusing, because I remember someone saying: you know, your ship may come in one day but sometimes you might just have to swim out a little to actually get it. And that's what we've got to do. We've got to swim out a bit.
>
> (Environmental health manager ID37, site 10)

It appears that whilst the majority of the factors leading to invisibility are perceived as being external, there are also internal factors around developing a more outward looking approach and taking steps to actively engage with local public health communities which would support the profession in playing a greater role in local government policymaking.

Understandings of environmental health

During interviews where the issue of invisibility arose, people were asked why they thought this was the case. There were a variety of suggestions, including the name, fragmentation and lack of clarity in the role, organisational structures and the domination of health and social care forcing other issues off policy agendas.

As I discussed in Chapter 2, the name of the occupation currently called environmental health has changed several times during its long history. With the benefit of hindsight, there was much regret expressed by some interviewees at the most recent name change from 'public health' (the term being first used in 1956) to 'environmental health' in 1974 (Cornell 1996), and it was widely felt that the loss of this simple flag of the primary role has affected how the occupation is perceived by others in the arena:

> People don't think of environmental health as a public health thing, strangely enough, and that's probably because the profession chose to call it environmental health rather than public health, which I think in retrospect is a mistake. I think it is public health and that would have focused people's minds on what it is about, so I think it is our own doing largely.
>
> (Environmental health manager ID32, site 5)

One interviewee was satisfied that they had retained the public health title for their service and felt that this was helpful:

> ...we wanted to make it very clear at the start that the title of the services is not Regulatory Services or Environmental Health – it's Public Health and Protection – so the fact you've got Public Health within the title of the Service... I often am aligned and speak with the drift of Public Health.
>
> (Environmental health manager ID34, site 7)

Many practitioners and managers expressed the view that environmental health was part of public health and felt no doubt that they have a vital role in the new system, even if this was invisible to others in that system:

> So the minimum amount of problems with your house, the minimum amount of noise and chemicals that you should be exposed to at work, and the likelihood that you're going to be killed or lose your foot or these kind of things, and I think we are quite vital. It's quite a vital role, but it is quite unseen I think.
>
> (Environmental health practitioner ID45, site 16; my emphasis)
>
> ...to my mind, fundamental to Environmental Health, because we are not Environmental Health, but Public Health, in my opinion. You know, if we're not involved in that, if we're not part of the process, then there's something seriously wrong with it.
>
> (Environmental health manager ID36, site 9)

It does appear that, in retrospect, the change in title from public health to environmental health was perhaps unhelpful, as practitioners now find themselves in a system where establishing public health credentials seems to be key to gaining recognition and playing a full role. However, the retention of the name would have necessitated a different title for the arm of public health that returned to the NHS; perhaps a 'healthcare public health' and 'local government public health' distinction would have been possible, reflecting the complementary and interconnected roles.

Many environmental health interviewees expressed the fragmentation of functions as an issue in the loss of identity and recognition by others; others suggested a lack of clarity around the environmental health role as a factor:

> ...environmental health practitioners have prided themselves on the fact that, you know, we're a jack of all trades and a master of none and we're always the meat in the sandwich, we are the people who put you in touch with other people, but I also think that doesn't sometimes be recognised as adding value.
>
> (Environmental health practitioner ID24, site 4)

> I think, we fragmented, we've lost some of that identity and, I think, therefore ... we're less easy to understand by people observing us and looking at us, an environmental health officer to one person, could be, 'oh, he's a noise officer, isn't he?'
>
> (Environmental health manager ID41, site 12)

Several interviewees suggested that the current difficulties have been largely self-inflicted, for example, tolerating poor practice:

> I've seen some dreadful environmental health officers, in my time, I've seen some good ones, but I've seen some dreadful ones and we don't do ourselves a lot of favours sometimes.
>
> (Environmental health manager ID41, site 12)

There was also some concern that the profession has lost its higher level strategic status by focusing primarily on technical issues:

> Public health is lost in the NHS and, as a profession, [we] never really got it back, not really fought for it back either – because we were too busy doing, you know, closing food premises down, and things like that, and dealing with more technical issues, so, I think, we lost our way as a profession.
>
> (Environmental health manager ID41, site 12)

There were issues around the impact of structural arrangements; some interviewees felt that fragmented or 'siloed' local regulatory organisational arrangements were potentially confusing in establishing a clear identity and visibility. Many environmental health interviewees mentioned that housing and other functions were part of a different department:

> ...different Councils do it differently, so you can have an Antisocial Behaviour Unit that's nothing to do with Environmental Health, that stuff like that would get shunted across to, once it gets to that stage and then [at] another Council, it would be the Environmental Health Officer all the way.
> (Environmental health practitioner ID45, site 16)

Some also felt that the profession was being lost amongst other functions in large directorates and noted a disconnect between regulatory occupations such as environmental health, trading standards and licensing. Others felt that not being located in the same department as the statutory public health policymaker was a disadvantage which had resulted in the service being overlooked:

> I was under the same department as head of policy, or if I was in the same department, or was in the Public Health Department, or I was with adult social care, if we were closely involved with the public health policymaking group, I think, that work would be recognised...
> (Environmental health manager ID31, site 4)

The Chartered Institute of Environmental Health is the national body for environmental health; however, many choose not to join. There is no requirement for practitioners to publish and no annual scientific conference to act as a vehicle for disseminating research within and outside the profession. With regard to the policymaking groups, the organisation had developed some publications nationally and campaigned at a high level for recognition; however, the impact did not appear to be felt locally. There also were some concerns regarding weak environmental health representation at a national level being a factor in visibility when compared to other occupational groups:

> I think, there doesn't seem to be that national voice either, because when I was doing the joint strategic needs assessment, the housing, the National Housing Agencies and the forums that housing was supposed to link into had a really strong voice about housing is really crucial ... had a huge evidence base around housing

interventions, we've got RSL, lobbying and saying it's wrong that we're not on the board ... but it just didn't seem to be there with Environmental Health.

(Public health policymaker support officer ID30, site 4)

The Chartered Institute seems to have been quiet, and there are publications there, because they have produced publications because I've seen them. But they don't seem to be ramming them down people's throats like other people do. I think there's been a lot of lobbying, and it doesn't feel as if they've done as much lobbying.

(Public health policymaker ID11, site 2)

These observations tended to come from those with non-environmental health backgrounds working within the wider public health arena, perhaps as they had the benefit of noting how different occupations responded to challenges in the new system. It is unclear why similar views were not so widely expressed by practitioners and managers, although it could be due to differences in experiences and expectations of what professional bodies can achieve on behalf of their members.

Challenges in becoming visible

It was also felt by many respondents that environmental health was generally suffering as a result of local authority budget cuts and that this was having an impact on the service, contributing to the loss of clarity and focus which was also expressed by others:

...it seems to me that the districts and boroughs are downgrading their environmental health services, which is a concern and I think that's happening right across the country, partly with the cuts and partly because of a lack of focus on what environmental health does.

(Public health policymaker ID15, site 1)

Some interviewees felt that the national policy emphasis on health and social care had overshadowed other functions with public health impacts:

...there's a massive expectation that social care and the health world can get together and solve a load of efficiency savings and duplication ... the implications for that for environmental health?

It puts ... some of those environmental health things into, you know, actually that's not that important at the moment.
(Environmental health manager ID34, site 7)

This suggestion is strongly supported by observational data, which shows health and social care issues dominating public health policy-maker agendas and meetings over a period of 18 months at all four case study sites – in particular, local arrangements for integrated health and social care. Site 1, for example, held an additional meeting to host a nationally recognised speaker with a particular interest in integrated care. There was a strong feeling in subsequent meetings at this site that the messages of this speaker had been taken on board and that integrated care was a priority locally. An interviewee had recognised that environmental health was being overlooked but was unclear why:

They [public health policymakers] probably naturally would select nurses and social workers and blah, blah, blah but what about environmental health? Why does this keep getting forgotten so much of the time? And I'm not quite sure why it is really.
(Environmental health practitioner and academic ID42)

Although, as I have described, there were many ideas put forward about why environmental health is invisible, environmental health practitioners and managers often could not understand why their role in tackling the social determinants of health was so unappreciated by others in the public health.

In overcoming invisibility, many environmental health interviewees mentioned the need to 'shout louder' or 'bang on the door' to make their voices heard in the new public health system to improve their visibility:

I am Chair of the [area] Chief Officers Group and so within that group I know that there was some frustration by Local Authorities, trying to find a way in... but as Chair I was able to write to various different people within the old [healthcare] structure and public health and just keep banging on the door and saying 'look, we're here and you need us'.
(Environmental health manager ID37, site 10)

This view was endorsed by public health policymaker support officers, who had noticed an absence of environmental health door-banging in some areas, often in contrast to other occupational groups such as housing managers and pharmacists:

> They're not knocking on the door saying 'why haven't we got a seat' [on the public health policymaking board] ... and whether the Environmental Health Officers are happy that their districts are represented at the level below, at the [area] board, I don't know, but I'd have expected them to be banging a lot harder on the door.
> (Public health policymaker ID11, site 2)

This need for specialists to 'be noisy and build alliances' has also been noted by others commenting on the current state of public health in England (Lang and Rayner 2012: 4), and it is possible that the absence of a university environmental health base or 'home' as a centre of excellence with clear links to the practitioner community and platform to hold conferences and raise issues is a contributory factor in the invisibility phenomenon. We are attempting to fill this gap at the University of Birmingham, but change takes time and requires broad cooperation and commitment beyond the institution.

Some managers had found a local focus on Marmot useful in promoting their service as having a role in tackling the social determinants of health. Others felt that environmental health managers needed to identify how their role fitted with the priorities of local policymakers in tackling health inequalities;

An environmental health manager (ID3, site 3), who was a member of an operational subgroup responsible for implementing Marmot principles, felt that the role offered many opportunities to demonstrate at a high level how their service could offer a practical public health input. A different environmental health manager at the same site explained how they had used Marmot to compile a report demonstrating their impact to the public health policymaker at a practical level, also recognising other local authority services and healthcare colleagues as having an existing role in tackling the social determinants of health:

> ...[it] really give examples of what we do within regulation enforcement that fit into each of the Marmot objectives, with a view obviously to trying to get an understanding of what we do in terms of our work to do with public health generally and reducing health inequalities across the board, but obviously we're only part of that and there is so much that goes on across the council and within the NHS public health, I think that the trick for the public health policymaking board

as it will be is to pull these things together and you can't do that unless you have a fair amount of knowledge about what goes on ...
(Environmental health manager ID4, site 3)

Another environmental health manager described how and why the involvement of environmental health had changed at their authority and also felt the need to recognise the role of other local authority services and to set out how joint working would happen in practice:

...when I arrived, I was quite shocked to find that environmental health was not part of this whole drive to tackle health inequalities, partly because ... I think, we had a head of services then who was not really engaged in the agenda... [and] as a profession as well that has, over the last few decades, found itself increasingly going down the regulatory route... so the County have said, look, we recognise that you are delivering a lot of public health at a local level through your environmental health teams, your housing teams, through your leisure services, your regulatory side, your licensing, housing advisor, homelessness, you know, we do an awful lot of public health here, not necessarily called environmental health, so they're saying, we recognise that and we need to agree with you how we're going to work together.
(Environmental health manager ID41, site 12)

An environmental health manager hoped for more recognition of the achievements and future potential of the profession, including in the relationships with local businesses:

...what I would like to see for environmental health is a better recognition of what we do to some of the priority areas, an example... we were instrumental in developing supplementary planning guidance that reduced the proliferation of hot food takeaways in certain parts of the borough and close to schools, it was something we got up, we provided the evidence base, we provided a monitoring mechanism for the planning service ... yet, we never get any recognition for all that groundwork which we did ..., we've got a better commercial interface with local businesses than anybody and we're in them regularly, we know where they are, we know who the key contacts are, they trust us and ... we're in a position of influence like, perhaps, nobody else within neither the [health service] or the Local Authority.
(Environmental health manager ID3, site 3)

An environmental health manager (ID43, site 14) who had success-fully made a case for funding from the health service to tackle health inequalities via a housing improvement programme felt that Marmot objectives had helped them to demonstrate their impact during pro-ject negotiations and discussion of outcome measures. There are sim-ilarities and differences in the enactment in policies and practice of environmental health relation to health inequalities. Some managers felt that Marmot had provided a useful framework to demonstrate impact, whereas at one context site in particular the situation was muddled.

As I have described in earlier chapters, the statutory public health policymaking group membership, wording of the enabling legisla-tion and much of the literature and available guidance places an emphasis on health and social care, and this is reflected in the meet-ing agendas. Some interviewees felt that this emphasis on health and social care had overshadowed other functions with public health impacts:

> ...there's a massive expectation that social care and the health world can get together and solve a load of efficiency savings and duplication ... the implications for that for environmental health? It puts ... some of those environmental health things into, you know, actually that's not that important at the moment.
> (Environmental health manager ID34, site 7)

Although, as I have described, there were many ideas put forward about why environmental health is invisible, practitioners and managers often could not understand why their role in tackling the social determinants of health was so unappreciated by others in the public health system.

There were serious concerns expressed by several people about the future of environmental health being under threat, being doubly invisible and under-recognised in the public health system, coupled with the negative effects of local authority spending cuts:

> And in better financial times Environmental Health Officers have been much more involved in terms of having much more health promotion type posts, but not being a statutory function, I think those tend to go when times get hard. So I don't know, and I sup-pose my sense is environmental health sort of retrenches to statu-tory functions when finances are tight.
> (Public health policymaker ID11, site 2)

Others felt that the new arrangements offered opportunities as well as threats:

> My own view is, if you don't embrace the opportunity, you are going to end up fighting with your existence in the not too distant future. So it's about, you know, we haven't got any choice and why would we want any choice actually, there's an opportunity here, there's an opportunity to make a real difference, let's grasp this.
> (Environmental health manager ID47, site 18)

An interviewee added that they felt recognition was improving, but that it would be a slow process:

> Environmental health practitioners are enormously powerful, it's an enormously powerful role and you think about what you can do in people's lives that no other profession, well other than perhaps acute medicine at that very urgent level can do, but when you think about the effect you could have on people's home life particularly, it's enormously, can be life changing – but it doesn't seem to be recognised for that, so I think there needs to be more work in that area. But I do think things are starting to shift, but it will be a long, uphill journey.
> (Environmental health practitioner and academic ID42)

References

Cornell, S. J. (1996). "Do environmental health officers practise public health?" *Public Health* 110(2): 73–75.

Lang, T. and G. Rayner (2012). "Ecological public health: the 21st century's big idea?" BMJ 345: e5466.

Rayner, G. and T. Lang (2012). *Ecological public health: Reshaping the conditions for good health*. London, Routledge.

6 The future of environmental health in public health

'Thinkers' and 'doers'

Environmental health practitioners and managers have observed that statutory functions are being lost, and new skills in securing funding are required to thrive in the new system, including being able to provide evidence of outcomes. I have found that environmental health practitioners see themselves as 'doers', compared to other public health colleagues as 'thinkers', and the role of evidence is key in this perception:

> ...the thing that I have in the back of my mind is people in the NHS seem to be very fixated with evidence based practice and, of course, environmental health, we just do it...
>
> (Environmental health manager ID1, site 3)

Several interviewees reported that the combination of expectation for evidence-based practice and lack of evidence in environmental health had caused tensions with public health colleagues, with one interviewee noting that the evidence base is 'like a religion in medicine' (Environmental health manager ID40, site 11). Others described the medical expectation to follow evidence-based practice as a potential cause of delays in decision-making for issues which require fast responses and had found this to be frustrating, again reinforcing the environmental health practitioner idea of themselves as 'doers' compared to other public health occupations:

> ...sometimes [there] has been a very good reason for the medical side to be very slow moving, very cautious ... whereas we sometimes have to be quite rapid and say I really want a bit of work done around this – will you draw me up a quick bit of policy and strategy for this and let's see if we can get something in place within the next three months?
>
> (Environmental health manager ID46, site 17)

One interviewee described a particularly uncomfortable situation in a meeting with public health colleagues when they questioned the use of the medical evidence-based practice norm to secure environmental health funding:

> But I also asked him, at this same meeting [laughing] – are you going to expect everybody that wants funding to provide you with an evidence based case, for why they require the funding and he looked at me like I was insane for even supposing that that wouldn't be needed.
>
> (Environmental health practitioner ID45, site 16)

Others alluded to a skills gap in terms of developing and using an evidence base in environmental health, but this was mentioned infrequently and indirectly. There was some hope expressed by several people that the relocation of public health colleagues to local authorities would provide a combined skill set that would help plug the evidence gap in environmental health:

> ...if we can make use of analysts, statisticians that are coming in from maybe from the PCT we then, possibly, [will] be in a better position to start contributing better and making a stronger argument when it comes to looking at priorities.
>
> (Environmental health manager ID31, site 4)

However, an environmental health manager expressed concerns that the move back to local authorities would lead to a loss of access to the evidence by colleagues formerly based in the National Health Service (NHS):

> ...where there is evidence they've got their finger on the pulse and I think we've not been particularly good at within the local authority is we're good at describing numbers in terms of what we do ... that's still a challenge for us and I'm hoping that we can learn from the NHS, but interestingly... they're worried by coming over, moving the public health stuff over to local authority they will lose those links and so that whereas now within the NHS they can you know they can go to somebody and say 'ooh well can you tell me what the obesity rates are in all the wards in [area]', if they're not working for them, those links may diminish and I so I think that that would be a challenge, but in terms of where they get information from and how they present it, they are streets ahead of us, I mean we can learn from that.
>
> (Environmental health manager ID4, site 3)

My research indicates that there is an expectation that evidence-based practice will be the norm for public health practitioners. Many environmental health interviewees reported experiences of evidence-based practice starting to dominate local expectations of public health practice, with environmental health struggling to demonstrate its value in these terms:

> Because, of course, that's the way that the NHS works. You can't get funding for any project or anything without having an evidence base behind it, which, of course, environmental health doesn't traditionally have ... and for example – why do we do food inspections? Where is the evidence base that they succeed or are worth funding?
>
> (Environmental health practitioner ID45, site 16)

The availability of evidence of outcomes rather than outputs in terms of inspections or other interventions is felt to be necessary to secure funding, if services (and ultimately jobs) are to be protected:

> We've barely scratched the surface of the analytics of some of the tobacco work, [but] we've actually got reasonable numbers about what we're doing. But big questions about does enforcement influence price? Does it influence availability? What will an elected member get for their money? If they give us another enforcement officer will there be measurable health impact? Are we just a finger in the dam wall and the best we can say is it's not getting any worse or are we actually making a difference? If we can actually show a meaningful cause and effect in terms of outcomes for say tobacco work I think the balance of spending from that would be different.
>
> (Environmental health manager ID46, site 17)

The environmental health profession does not have a tradition of evidence-based or evidence-informed practice, and this is the case both in using the available evidence for decision-making (including accessing it) and evaluating and writing up work to contribute to the development of an evidence base. An example of an attempt at evidence-based practice was the introduction of the Housing Health and Safety Rating System in 2006, which used the available evidence to generate a risk-based approach to housing enforcement interventions. The operating guidance for the system requires users to consider the best available evidence; however, in practice, there is a reliance on the now out-of-date guidance. This shows that even where evidence is available, there is a need for systems to be in place to ensure it is updated in order for practitioners to access and use it appropriately.

Many environmental health interviewees reported feeling unable to provide the evidence required of them in the new public health system:

> ...there's lots of information out there to say what the problems are, but to prove that what you did had an impact, is very difficult, and because it's evidence based, everyone's looking for you to prove it. So, that is tricky.
> (Environmental health manager ID36, site 9)

Other interviewees agreed that they had encountered difficulties in measuring the outcomes of environmental health work, which is primarily preventative. One environmental health manager reported challenges in negotiating for time to measure longer-term outcomes in a system where short-term outcomes are of greater interest, giving an example of issues arising during a smoking cessation project:

> ...it was a battle to get the money and it was a battle to stop it getting shat on (pardon me) by the Performance Manager at the PCT. It was a battle to get people to keep their faith when nothing's happened. You know, you've been doing it for six months and nothing's happened.
> (Environmental health manager ID40, site 11)

Many environmental health managers shared these difficulties in measuring the public health outcomes for their services, feeling that relying on less tangible outputs as a measurement of effectiveness was rendering them vulnerable to a loss of resources:

> ...if your service is doing well and you don't have the numbers of prosecutions and notices served, or homelessness cases, you know, there's a temptation for the members to think that there's too much capacity in those areas, they're thinking, well, there isn't a problem, therefore, we don't need so many staff, but it's actually the front line work that's going on that's preventing that kind of thing.
> (Environmental health manager ID35, site 8)

Others felt that the environmental health experience was also true for other local government occupations:

> ...we do a project and it often is pretty good, but we don't necessarily review it, we don't document it ... we have some outcomes, but most often they are usually figures, aren't they? They're not... what have we actually achieved from a public health point of view and we don't share it very often ... But then I don't necessarily think we're on our own within local government being like that.
>
> (Environmental health manager ID1, site 3; my emphasis)

There are mixed feelings about what the future looks like for environmental health, but there is a feeling that if visibility is to improve it will require significant effort on the part of practitioners, managers and at the national level to raise the profile with allied groups and policymakers.

Evidence-based practice

Evidence-based policy and practice have become increasingly important ideas in medicine and public health. Cookson (2005: 119) provides a useful differentiation between evidence-based medicine and evidence-based policy (in healthcare) whilst recognising that they are similar concepts. He defines evidence-based policymaking as that which 'focuses on public policy decisions about groups of people rather than decisions about individual patients'. Using this definition, it could be argued that evidence-based public health is strongly related to evidence-based policy in general, since the discipline is concerned with populations rather than individuals.

Qualitative approaches in research can be useful when developing evidence-based policy: several academics (Pollitt, Harrison et al. 1990; Cookson 2005) have commented on the need for a qualitative approach when researching policy, where randomised controlled trials and other 'experiments' are not possible. However, qualitative research may not be designed to influence policymaking, with some academics making clear that the main aim of their work is not to make 'practical recommendations for action' (Pollitt, Harrison et al. 1990: 182) and research may not be written in a 'user friendly' way for practitioners to utilise. Others have found a general lack of assessment of health technology in public health and speculate that this could be because 'they are inherently more complex ... [and] ... are usually multisectoral, politically charged and often considered mundane and "common sense" and, thus, not requiring evaluation' (Holland 2004: 77). What follows is that accessing research, drawing conclusions and making generalisations for use in future policymaking is not straightforward; creating an evidence base for policymaking and public health is trickier than creating one for medicine. However, Stuckler and Basu (2013) argue that evaluating public policies is vital for effective and informed democratic decision-making.

Even where there is evidence for policymaking, it has been found that 'there is a considerable gap between what research shows is effective and the policies that are enacted and enforced', and Brownson et al. (2009: 1576–1577) go on to identify eight 'barriers to implementing effective public health policy':

- Lack of value placed on prevention
- Insufficient evidence base
- Mismatched time horizons
- Power of vested interests
- Researchers isolated from the policy process
- Policy process can be complex and messy
- Individuals in any one discipline may not understand the policy-making process as a whole
- Practitioners lack the skills to influence evidence-based policy.

Marks (2006) adds that similar barriers exist in using evidence to tackle health inequalities, citing a lack of evidence, ongoing theoretical debates and the type of evidence (avoiding focusing on simplistic, easy to measure issues) as important considerations.

An additional challenge is that public health interventions often require a long-term commitment, for which progress can be difficult to measure in the shorter term, and that expectations for results in a given time period can be unrealistic (Bauld and Judge 2008). Jo Webber, deputy policy director of the NHS Confederation, summed these difficulties up in her evidence to the Health Select Committee:

> There are some proxies you could use for the short-term – and by short-term I am meaning one, two or three years – but, with some public health interventions, it is going to take you 10 or 20 years before you see what that outcome might be, by which time you are going to have had probably two or three changes of idea about which way this is all going. Therefore, it is about getting the right

proxies in place as well in the short term and then allowing the evidence base to be built.

(House of Commons Health Committee 2011)

Greenhalgh and Russell (2009: 310) argue that an evidence-based policy approach will not identify 'what the right policy is for every particular situation', as this depends upon the judgements made in framing 'the problem'. They say that 'political problems are turned into technical ones, with the concomitant danger that political programmes are disguised as science' and others note that, with regard to Health Action Zones, 'early wins' were targeted for political expediency (Bauld and Judge 2008). Rayner (2007: 454) adds that a new approach to public health is needed '…beyond the timid evidence based perspective', going on to say that evidence is useful but needs to be seen as a resource rather than a limitation, and Tannahill (2008) promotes 'making decisions in good faith' which recognises the roles of evidence, theory and ethics in public health decision-making. These observations are extremely pertinent to the emphasis on local democracy in the current political agenda, the development of strategies of public health policymakers to tackle health inequalities and the position of environmental health.

Observers have recently noted that linking funding for health promotion activities to evidence-based practice is 'now the norm' (Dunne, Scriven et al. 2012); however, they raise concerns that the evaluation of work to create evidence which informs future work requires investment. They also note, as I have described earlier, that evaluating health promotion initiatives is not straightforward and that medical 'gold standard' approaches such as the randomised controlled trial cannot be utilised in many community situations.

Scriven (2012: 108) asks 'what counts as evidence and what methods are appropriate in measuring intervention effectiveness?' These are potentially important issues for the future of environmental health. Others consider that 'what is counted as evidence, and methods for gathering and synthesising evidence, will need to be substantially broadened' (Marks 2002: 44). A survey of people working in public health found that there were concerns of bias in evidence, different understandings of what constitutes evidence and issues around access to resources (UK Health Forum 2013). The access issue is very real for local authority-based occupations, as traditionally local authorities have not subscribed to services allowing access to peer-reviewed journals (Couch, Stewart et al. 2012). There are some hopes that this will change as a result of the relocation of formally NHS-based public health practitioners, who would have had access in their previous roles and would expect this to continue. The emphasis on open access publication should also improve the situation for local government based practitioners.

The UK Environmental Health Research Network (EHRNet), of which I am a founder member, has defined evidence-based environmental health as

>...environmental health policy and practice supported by the best available evidence, taking into account the preferences of citizens and the wider public and our own professional judgment.
>
>(Barratt, Couch et al. 2013: 2)

Evidence-based practice, as I have discussed in Chapter 1, has become a medical norm in rhetoric, if not always in practice. Whilst this has been established in medicine for some time, it has not been true for local government occupations, where local strategic decision-making has been the prerogative of elected members, advised by officers who do not have a tradition of evidence-based practice. This is not to say that the idea of evidence-based practice in environmental health and other local government professions has been dismissed historically; however, it never became established as an expectation of good practice, as one interviewee recalled:

>...I can remember when I was at college in the mid-eighties, our head of course at Leeds, was then saying, Environmental Health has to be better at evaluating the projects it does and saying how good it is. And we're still not good at that.
>
>(Environmental health manager ID44, site 15)

Interviews with environmental health practitioners and managers have revealed both individuals and the wider body struggling to accept the need for and the practicalities of adapting to an evidence-based practice approach in order to survive and establish some credibility in the new system. There is also some evidence to suggest that other local government occupational groups such as social workers find themselves in a similar situation (Fronek 2013).

There was general agreement that environmental health practitioners were carrying out a lot of good, effective work, but were failing to evaluate, write up and publish in order to develop the evidence base now required:

>...the reality is there's people out there experimenting every day of their life, but they don't realise they're doing it, and they're not recording it, well they're not doing it in an appropriate way perhaps,

but they're not recording it either, and they're not sharing, except in anecdotes.

(Environmental health practitioner with national role ID33)

There also appears to be an expectation from public health colleagues that evidence will be quantitative or 'medical':

> ...what I see in terms of what evidence will be used to make decisions and, without a doubt, most of it is medical; there is still a lack of environmental/social evidence, I think that is of higher status, if you like and, and powerful enough to affect decisions ... it is much easier to churn out some of the medical data more quickly and some professions have much more of a culture of that than others. So I think that is going to be quite a stumbling block, particularly if people have to fight their way in, rather than, are welcomed in on an equal footing.
>
> (Environmental health practitioner and academic ID42)

It can be seen that there is not simply an issue with a lack of evidence: the type of evidence and the way it is presented is seen as crucial in being accepted as a public health profession of legitimacy and value. There were very real concerns reported about the impact of a lack of evidence-based practice in environmental health and the consequent inability to present the available data effectively inhibiting engagement as equals in the new public health system:

> ...unfortunately, well fortunately or unfortunately, fortunately the public health in the NHS, they do that very well ... So I think there's a danger we've got there of not being able to be part of it ... I think the only way we are going to prove ourselves, is, is by the results we give and that's how I go back to measuring stuff... because it's very hard to go to these meetings when they've got massive graphs and it's all very well presented and we turn up with 'well we did all this' and it looks like a bit of scrap of paper, so it's how we present ourselves, how we get ourselves on a level playing field really.
>
> (Environmental health manager ID1, site 3)

One interviewee took this concern a step further, by identifying the risk that environmental health would lose out to more organised 'others':

...the people who are good at that may get ahead of us in the queue and we'll still be going: You can't cut this. You can't cut this. This is so important.

(Environmental health manager ID46, site 17)

There were specific concerns that funding could be lost:

... there hasn't been the research done to be able to just go and find a paper that says: Environmental Health – this project should be funded – because it makes this much impact. That research doesn't exist – or it hasn't been published.

(Environmental health practitioner ID45, site 16)

Others were concerned that the lack of evidence could affect the ability of environmental health to engage effectively with public health policymakers:

...if we really want to have an impact on those Boards and in strategy and also make sure they've got the right resource it's to have – you have to have the right research and the background to prove your case.

(Environmental health manager ID34, site 7)

This research has found that the need for evidence has added a layer of complexity, and sometimes tension, between occupational groups, as they are required to cooperate but may also be competing for limited funding. Nevertheless, there is optimism that many issues can be overcome by working more closely together, learning from others and playing to their relative strengths.

Using evidence and other strategies for impact

As I have discussed elsewhere (Dhesi and Stewart 2015), many environmental health practitioners and managers expressed the view that the historic focus on outputs rather than outcomes was proving unhelpful and regretted measurement of the job role and impact by other bodies in this way (such as the Food Standards Agency for food hygiene inspections) had not been challenged earlier:

...we've, sort of, allowed ourselves, as a profession... to be measured by the number of inspections we did, how quickly we turned around, how many high risk, medium, low risk and the same with health and safety. So we should have been more robust in challenging that, you know, we were, when we started out at, as a profession, we were very challenging.

(Environmental health manager ID41, site 12)

An environmental health manager expanded this theme, adding that outputs measured were often targeted at the wrong issues:

We wanted to be a risk based/intelligence based service. That means we are trying to move from being output based – how many inspections do you do? So what? What difference does it make? Even if you're fully compliant with the Food Standards Agency requirements, so what? We're trying to get to the point where we've got enough intelligence and needs assessment generally to be able to start challenging. Why are we doing all of those inspections when we should look at the size of the issues – is it food poisoning or is it obesity?

(Environmental health manager ID34, site 7)

One interviewee felt that the Chartered Institute of Environmental Health (CIEH), the national body for environmental health, had been remiss in not establishing evidence-based practice historically:

I think it comes back to the thing about evidence and we haven't got the evidence as a profession and that's our own fault really, but I think the CIEH hasn't been as rigorous as might have been in that respect.

(Environmental health practitioner and academic ID42)

Despite this, several interviewees reported negative experiences of evidence-based practice and felt that in practice the concept was limiting in terms of innovation in dealing with novel problems, obtaining funds for pioneering work and ensuring a speedy response:

one thing I would say about NHS public health officers is that they're very good at justifying what they do and I've had a few shall we say interesting discussions because they, they're always going on about everything's got to be evidence based and I do understand that that's important but there are times when you haven't got the evidence, you can't get the evidence, for instance the work that [we've] done with sheesha, this has been unique, if we'd scratched around trying to find some evidence that it's a good idea to go into a sheesha premises and stop them operating illegally, well, we'd still be examining our navels quite frankly, sometimes you just have to go there and get on with it and interestingly some of the NHS colleagues have agreed with that view.

(Environmental health manager ID4, site 3)

One interviewee expressed concerns that evidence-based practice was being used in a very limited way, resulting in a backwards focus:

We only know about what we have been doing, we don't even research that well enough but we certainly don't research what we could be doing – and so everybody who is looking at the evidence base is looking for the things they are already doing, well that's a distortion we can't live with.

(Environmental health practitioner with national role ID33)

This suggests the view that evidence-based practice was a good thing in itself was clearly not universally held.

When asked about why environmental health did not have a tradition of evidence-based practice, a variety of ideas were suggested, although by far the most common response was lack of time, often related to how they were currently measured in their role:

...if your job is to do that and to crunch out the statistics, because that's what it comes down to, how do you then find the time and the energy to do the things that actually might be more important and have more of an impact on health?

(Environmental health practitioner and academic ID42)

A practitioner, who appreciated the need to create and use an evidence base, when comparing environmental health with other public health colleagues, felt that the time issue must be overcome:

One of the things that really shook me was I, I spent a couple of days working for the Health Protection Agency, and I noticed how good they are at evidencing what they do... when you read their monthly report book ... it's just so professionally done ... and you think well, should we be getting more serious about that in Environmental Health? I think we probably should be ... that we do seem to be too often just sort of chasing our

tails round, setting fixed penalties for littering when we should
be looking at (I'm not belittling what we do on a day to day
basis) but there should be some time put aside to do these types
of projects.

(Environmental health practitioner ID38, site 10)

An environmental health manager considered evidence-based practice a 'luxury' rather than a necessity, where resources are tight, but
had hopes for future working with public health colleagues following
their relocation:

We're a streamlined service, we don't have much fat on the makeup
of the teams and finding time to look into research, look into developing and building baseline data that you can work from is
something that we don't have the luxury of being able to do, that's
one of the things I'm hoping, public health coming in to local authorities might help us with.

(Environmental health manager ID31, site 4)

Interestingly, there was very little direct mention of a lack of skill
or confidence in being able to evaluate, write up and publish projects; this was surprising, given the high level of interest and their
perceived need to develop research skills seen in attendees at work-
shops on these topics organised by the UK Environmental Health
Research Network.

There were two notable success stories in the use of evidence-based
practice reported by environmental health manager interviewees,
both working in cities, though at different ends of the country and in
very different circumstances. The first relates to success in levering
in funding for housing interventions to tackle health inequalities, by
quantifying spend on environmental health and modelling for savings
in health and other public spending:

We've had very long debates about outcomes and outputs because you know these things are so difficult to measure, you
know if you're exposed to substandard housing the symptoms
may not manifest themselves for 5, 10, 15 years and there's no
way you can have a sort of impact assessment or evaluation done
in a short period of time, but what we are able to do is model ...
So Environmental Health Officers in year 1 cost roughly
£300,000 in salaries levered in by in terms of landlord improvements several hundred thousand pounds and will be saving, or

are estimated to save the NHS £4.4 million over 10 years and wider society £11 million.

(Environmental health manager ID43, site 14)

The second manager had used a variety of approaches to demonstrate the effectiveness of their service:

...we've done quite a bit of evidence based evaluation but it's been both qualitative and quantitative, so we have done quite a lot of feedback on a qualitative manner, so interviews as well as the nub of how many referrals, to whom and all that sort of stuff ... and it is quite difficult when you get asked; right, what are your outcomes, what are you monitoring to actually come up with something that's useable? Because we tend to deal with things over a longer term so it is quite difficult sometimes, but I think we're creative.

(Environmental health manager ID48, site 19)

These limited examples demonstrate that evidence-based practice or perhaps more accurately evidence-informed practice is possible in environmental health, that it is happening in some areas and also, perhaps more importantly, that it has been used effectively to protect and grow services following the recognition of the impact of the role.

Building on the success stories, there was some positivity expressed by interviewees around the practical steps that could be taken to start evaluating, giving sufficient thought to how success will be measured at the planning stage of a project:

So you're looking at it at the beginning going; right, okay, well, what do we want to achieve and how are we going to monitor it? Not doing it and then getting halfway through going; what have we done and what have we achieved, you really need to start at the beginning and do it then ...

(Environmental health manager ID48, site 19)

Others felt that being able to demonstrate the value of environmental health work would make an impact in how they are perceived:

If we do this and we show the benefits, then it's going to be a lot of benefit to us, because people will say, 'Well look, Environmental Health, they've really delivered here.

(Environmental health manager ID36, site 9)

Finally, an interviewee with a strategic role in local government expressed an openness to considering the value of broader non-medical evidence for public health:

> ...probably it's easier in housing where there was a bigger national evidence base... if ... the housing intervention costs a few hundred pounds, but could potentially save thousands of pounds in hospital treatment, that's where you actually do start getting people going, oh yeah, and then you can tie that back to the Joint Strategic Needs Assessment ... I think it's about normalising what you think of as public health.
>
> (Public health policymaker support officer ID30, site 4)

References

Barratt, C., R. Couch, A. Page, S. Dhesi, and J. Stewart (2013). *An Introduction to Evidence Based Environmental Health.* http://ukehrnet.wordpress.com/2013/09/11/research-briefing-1-introducing-evidence-based-eh/, UK Environmental Health Network (EHRNet).

Bauld, L. and K. Judge (2008). "Strong theory, flexible methods. Evaluating complex community-based initiatives." In *Critical Perspectives in Public Health.* Eds. J. Green and R. Labonte. London, Routledge: 93–103.

Brownson, R. C., J. F. Chriqui, and K. A. Stamatakis (2009). "Understanding evidence-based public health policy." *Government, Politics, and Law* 99(9): 1576–1583.

Cookson, R. (2005). "Evidence-based policy making in health care: what it is and what it isn't." *Journal of Health Services Research and Policy* 10(2): 118–121.

Couch, R., J. Stewart, C. Barratt, S. Dhesi, and A. Page (2012). *Evidence, Research and Publication: A Guide for Environmental Health Professionals.* E-book, Lulu.

Dhesi, S. and J. Stewart (2015). "The developing role of evidence-based environmental health: perceptions, experiences, and understandings from the front line." *SAGE Open* (September–December): 1–10.

Dunne, A., A. Scriven, and C. Furlong (2012). "Funding linked to evidence: what future for health promotion?" *Perspectives in Public Health* 132(3): 109–110.

Fronek, P. H. (2013). *Evidence-Based Practice: In Conversation with Debbie Plath.* Podsocs. Podcast www.podsocs.com/podcast/evidence-based-practice/. Griffith University.

Greenhalgh, T. and J. Russell (2009). "Evidence-based policymaking: a critique." *Perspectives in Biology and Medicine* 52(2): 304–318.

Holland, W. W. (2004). "Health technology assessment and public health: a commentary." *International Journal of Technology Assessment in Health Care* 20(1): 77–80.

House of Commons Health Committee (2011). *Corrected Transcript of Oral Evidence*, Tuesday 7 June 2011. H. C. House of Commons. London, House of Commons.

Marks, D. (2002). *Perspectives on Evidence-Based Practice*. London, Health Development Agency Public Health Evidence Steering Group.

Marks, L. (2006). "An evidence base for tackling inequalities in health: distraction or necessity?" *Critical Public Health* 16(1): 61–71.

Pollitt, C., S. Harrison, D. Hunter, and G. Marnoch (1990). "No hiding place: on the discomforts of researching the contemporary policy process." *Journal of Social Policy* 19(2): 169–190.

Rayner, G. (2007). "Multidisciplinary public health: Leading from the front?" *Public Health* 121(6): 449–454.

Scriven, A. (2012). "Guest editorial. Funding linked to evidence: what future for health promotion?" *Perspectives in Public Health* 132(3): 108.

Stuckler, D. and S. Basu (2013). *The Body Economic. Why Austerity Kills*. London, Allen Lane, Penguin Books.

Tannahill, A. (2008). "Beyond evidence – to ethics: a decision-making framework for health promotion, public health and health improvement." *Health Promotion International* 23(4): 380–390.

UK Health Forum (2013). *Evidence in Public Health: The Results from an Online Survey*. Available at http://www.ukhealthforum.org.uk/who-we-are/our-work/research-information-services/publications/?entryid43=42172&cord=ASC&p=3

7 Conclusions

By bringing together my research, lecturer and practitioner experiences, I hope that I have been able to offer some insight into the current position of the environmental health profession and how it is perceived by others working in related fields. By sharing my research findings in this accessible format, I also hope the evidence conveyed will secure necessary actions to maximise the potential for protecting and improving the public's health.

My findings suggest that the environmental health profession must *define* and, importantly, *communicate* what it stands for and what it can offer as a specialism as part of the broad public health workforce. A clear and easily recognisable identity is required. There is much misunderstanding and confusion amongst public health policymakers both in local government and beyond around the role and what environmental health practitioners can offer as contributors to a wider team. We can no longer assume that people understand what the role involves, and whilst there are some examples of recognition at local levels, a coordinated, national-level or even international-level effort appears to be required.

Environmental health practitioners also need to be open to working beyond narrow statutory functions and liaising with other professional groups sharing common or overlapping objectives. Statutory functions and measurements of success also need reviewing to ensure that efforts are targeted at areas with the greatest potential for impacting public health and tackling health inequalities. These developments should in turn bring funding opportunities, recognition, interest and variation into the role. However, policies of austerity have impacted the scale and scope of the local government workforce in many areas and this change will take time to embed.

These steps should also serve to increase the profile of the profession beyond the public health community and thus attract bright and ambitious new members to join. Many of our students at Birmingham have been drawn to the role by a professional encounter, for example, whilst working in the food industry or in other local authority departments; very few appear to have made the decision to study environmental health without a direct introduction, recommendation or experience. This indicates that opportunities to recruit to the profession are being lost.

The Chartered Institute of Environmental Health has a role to play in making this happen, and my findings indicate that a clear and coherent message from the organisation was not heard at policymaking levels at the crucial time. Whilst environmental health covers a very broad remit which can make communication challenging, other professional groups encompassing widely varied roles such as general practitioners, surveyors and engineers demonstrate that it is possible to link a broad range of specialisms together in a cohesive and recognisable professional identity.

Given the history of the profession and impacts of environmental health work in protecting the most vulnerable, it is my strongly held view that our professional identity must be linked to social justice and equity. The role in tackling health and other inequalities has been largely overlooked, and this should be reclaimed as central to our ethos.

My research strongly indicates that environmental health as a profession is suffering from double invisibility, in that public health is culturally invisible, and within this, environmental health is invisible. Practitioners and managers expressed difficulties in promoting their service to decision makers, their allied occupational groups and elected members, and a variety of reasons were given for this. It appears that the exclusion of environmental health from the statutory list of public health policymaking group members has been unhelpful, in that health and social care issues have taken precedence, with environmental health seen as one amongst many other groups vying for attention.

As I have described, this double invisibility is strongly felt by practitioners and managers, who consider their service vital. However, this sense of importance does not appear to be shared by the majority of public health policymakers, support officers and other allied public health occupations, particularly those involved in setting local policies and strategies.

Moving onto environmental health practice, my research suggests that the evidence-based practice is fast becoming the expectation across the public health system. This reality has caused problems for local government public health occupations, such as environmental health, that are not geared up to evidence their work in terms of outcomes, having historically been measured by external bodies (such as the Food Standards Agency) in terms of outputs such as the number of routine inspections carried out on time. This puts environmental health at a disadvantage when demonstrating its value as a public health occupation and, it is felt, may impact on service funding in the future.

My findings have shown that there are signs that environmental health practitioners and managers feel that by evaluating their work in terms of outcomes, they will be better able to demonstrate the benefits of their efforts. However, the nature of the work and timeframes involved can make this challenging, and proxy indicators may need to be explored.

Many environmental health practitioners and managers recognise the deficit in the use and generation of evidence, and whilst they may not all agree on the value of evidence-based practice in itself, they do see that being able to demonstrate effectiveness and value for money is necessary to survive and thrive. There is some optimism that this can be developed, particularly if efforts are made to work with other public health colleagues more familiar with the concept; however, there does not seem to be much willingness to compromise on the requirement for evidence-based practice by other (primarily medical) public health professional groups.

A further issue is the use of the existing and, in many specialisms such as air pollution, substantial evidence base to inform practice. This appears to be partly due to access issues – although open access publications are becoming commonplace and should improve this situation in time – and partly due to a lack of time and managerial acknowledgement of the value of taking evidence into account when planning interventions. The available evidence is also often in rather inaccessible formats, and some work is needed to bring new and relevant findings and their implications for practice to the attention of practitioners.

Looking to the role of academia, whilst there are academic research centres for environmental health in the UK, these tend to focus on specific areas, for example, air pollution at the University of Birmingham. However, we are lacking in a centre where environmental health is researched at a high level across its breadth and where there are strong links between the academic and practitioner communities, generating solid, useable outputs to impact practice. The few environmental health practitioner-researchers that do exist are generally employed in health or social services faculties or, alternatively, in law, housing or food faculties, depending upon their specialism and interests.

Environmental health practitioner-researchers remain rare, which was one of the drivers for establishing Environmental Health Network (EHRNet). This rarity may be linked to the practice of lecturers on environmental health courses being recruited for their practitioner skills rather than their research abilities or experience; consequently teaching departments do not often have a strong research base from which to teach students; to encourage and prepare them to contribute to environmental health research and publication once qualified; or to embark on doctoral study themselves. This would, in time, raise the visibility and status of environmental health with other public health groups and beyond.

In our teaching at the University of Birmingham, we emphasise the requirements for critical thinking, the value of peer-reviewed literature and the need for baseline and in-project evaluation in our teaching. However, we have found that our graduates encounter challenges and are frequently unable to follow this through in the workplace due to the time constraints and other pressures in their local government roles. We are ambitious for our graduates and hope that when they become managers and policymakers they will recall the benefits of these practices. We have made some inroads on closing the gaps between academia and practitioner communities, but there remains a great deal of work to be done. Engaging with research should be viewed as essential to professional life, not a piece of work to be delivered and then shelved in order to qualify to practice. However, funding and support, including academic library access, for joint impactful research remains an issue.

In my view, as a profession we must maintain a commitment to graduate-level education in environmental health, so whilst covering technical issues across the various specialisms, we also embed critical thinking, evidence-based practice, evaluation and publication in the professional expectations of the next generation, who will need the skills to become tomorrow's managers and leaders.

In addition, postgraduate routes, including doctoral study, need to be embraced and supported so as to be considered fairly routine career options, rather than an unusual pathway (as is currently the case). For this to happen, universities, if recruiting staff based on technical skills and experience, will need to support lecturers to undertake doctoral research when appointed. In time, this should build a critical mass of practitioner-academics equipped to develop and lead centres of excellence aimed at working with and supporting the practitioner community.

Finally, although it can be highly challenging, I have found combining life as an academic and practitioner to be very rewarding. One of the aims of writing this book was to highlight the benefits to practitioners and the wider profession of joining up research and practice and to encourage others to develop careers spanning these two worlds. This is the norm in many other health and public health fields, so why not environmental health?

Index

Milton Keynes UK
Ingram Content Group UK Ltd.
UKHW031137141024
449569UK00006B/114